BALANCE
TRAINING

BALANCE
T R A I N I N G
Stability Workouts for Core Strength and a Sculpted Body

KARON KARTER

Photography by **Andy Mogg**

Ulysses Press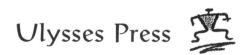

Published in the United States by Ulysses Press
P.O. Box 3440
Berkeley, CA 94703
www.ulyssespress.com

ISBN10: 1-56975-605-8
ISBN13: 978-1-56975-605-8
Library of Congress Control Number 2006938935

Printed in Canada by Webcom

10 9 8 7 6 5 4 3 2 1

Editorial/Production	Lily Chou, Claire Chun, Lisa Kester, Ruth Marcus, Matt Orendorff, Elyce Petker, Steven Zah Schwartz, Laurel Shane
Index	Sayre Van Young
Cover design	Matt Orendorff
Cover photographs	Andy Mogg
Models	Shani Compton, Kurt Johnson, Karon Karter, Toni Silver

Distributed by Publishers Group West

Please Note
This book has been written and published strictly for informational purposes, and in no way should be used as a substitute for consultation with health care professionals. You should not consider educational material herein to be the practice of medicine or to replace consultation with a physician or other medical practitioner. The author and publisher are providing you with information in this work so that you can have the knowledge and can choose, at your own risk, to act on that knowledge. The author and publisher also urge all readers to be aware of their health status and to consult health care professionals before beginning any health program.

To my mother

table of contents

acknowledgments

It takes a village to put a book together, and books often begin with an idea. I usually come up with my own idea, but not this time. Acquisitions editor Nick Denton-Brown tracked me down and trusted me to create a book based on Ulysses Press's vision—thank you so much. Thanks to Lily Chou and Claire Chun for being editors par excellence; they helped shape my words and do just about everything else to get the book into print. On the production and marketing end, Matt Orendorff, Steven Schwartz, Bryce Willett and Beth Cook worked to get the book into bookstores. Thank you, Marilyn Allen, for being the best kind of agent—patient, brilliant and oh-so-nice.

On the home front, thank you Luke's Locker (where I teach Pilates to my runners) for giving me cute outfits to wear during the photo shoot. And I'm grateful to photographer Andy Mogg, as well as models Toni Silver and Shani Compton, for making the photo shoot a breeze. I'm deeply indebted to Kurt Johnsen of American Power Yoga for not only being my male model and wonderful travel companion, but for giving me the opportunity of a lifetime. Of course, I would never be able to follow my dreams if it weren't for my family—I truly am a blessed girl!

—Karon Karter

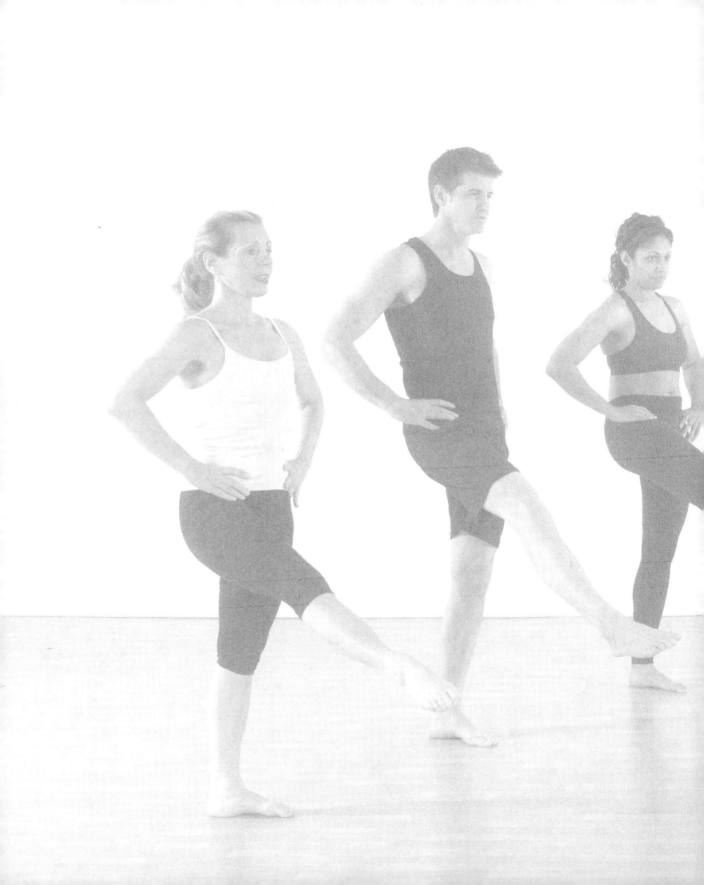

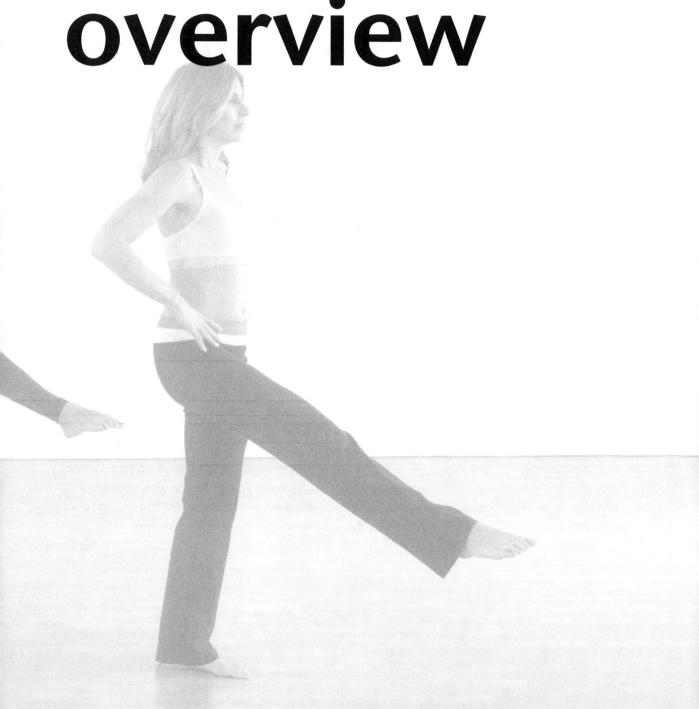

part one:
overview

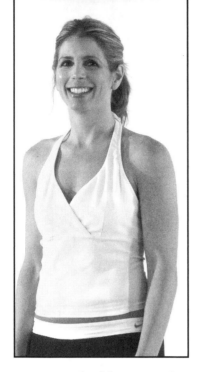

introduction

Dare to bare your legs, your super-toned tummy, or your bikini-clad bum? Well, good news! You'll love the way the stability workouts in *Balance Training* coordinate your entire musculature to achieve more balance, strength, and a stronger look overall. In other words, "Wow—I want your body fast!"

In everyday life, you rarely use one muscle at a time. You must call on a variety of muscles to keep you steady on your feet and to help you move. Even a simple movement such as walking recruits several muscles to get your legs moving. Balance and strength provide the foundation for all movement, so it's important to engage an array of muscles to closely duplicate your daily activities while incorporating stability and balance challenges at the same time. That's where these workouts come in. You'll be required to strike a pose over a dynamic, ever-changing surface to hone your balance skills and reap maximum strength and calorie-burning benefits. All of this results in a slimmer, stronger, and more stable you. Regardless of your fitness level, you can have the Wow! Body.

So what is balance? Can our bodies be balanced yet our lives out of balance? I often ask myself this question as I struggle to maintain balance in my own life. Here's what I do know: As a Pilates instructor, I'm always looking for balance in my clients' bodies. Inevitably, if their bodies are out of balance, then they hurt; minor aches and pains bring them down. However, if I can create balance in their bodies, then everything else seems to work itself out. It's not because I have some kind of miracle cure. Rather, it's because they don't have to waste precious energy worrying about their bodies. Simply, they feel good because balance feels good! I truly believe that balance begins with a healthy body— everything else falls into place.

balance in your body

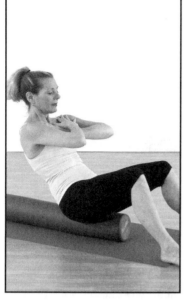

If you train only one way, you're training ineffectively. Of course, it's impossible to say what the best approach to training is, but if you cross-train in a manner designed to challenge all systems of your body and movement patterns, you'll have a healthier body overall. So, can stability workouts keep you fit and healthy? You bet!

The *Balance Training* workouts will enhance whatever fitness routine you may be doing by adding a cross-training element. Not only will you improve your balance, you'll increase your strength, especially core strength (meaning strong torso muscles), and tone up a variety of muscles. In addition, as your strength and stability improve, your daily movements will become more efficient.

According to the American College of Sports Medicine (ACSM), one of the world's largest exercise certifying bodies, your weekly fitness routine should include cardio, strength, and flexibility. You should be doing a combination of heart-pumping exercises, known as cardio, three days a week for 20–60 minutes a day, as well as strength exercises two to three days a week. This involves training and stretching each major muscle group at least two to three days a week. The workouts in this book go beyond the ACSM recommendations by including stability challenges and core-strength exercises, which are also vital fitness elements.

Anti-Aging Bonus

These days you can't turn on the television without hearing that Americans are living longer. The American Geriatrics Society reports that by 2030, the number of adults age 65 and older will nearly double to 70 million. There is little doubt that fitness functions as an anti-aging ingredient and improves quality of life. Even so, as the new sports medicine science of prevention expands to include research on baby boomers, you'll hear more about the benefits of balance and core-strength exercises.

Typically, balance happens automatically, or at least doesn't require you to think about it. In a healthy body, your senses (touch, sight, and hearing) work in harmony with your brain to help you balance. As you age, you may lose one or more of your senses in addition to muscle mass. Between the two, including the added effects of degenerative diseases, medications, and accumulated injuries such as ear infections, you can slowly lose the ability to balance.

Muscle contractions make up all physical movements while stability provides the foundation for movement. You can't get out of a chair, walk, jump, or bend over to tie your shoes without a combination of both strength and balance. If balance problems develop, you can disrupt every movement of your daily life and increase your risk of falls.

The good news is that you can train your balance, just like any other fitness element;

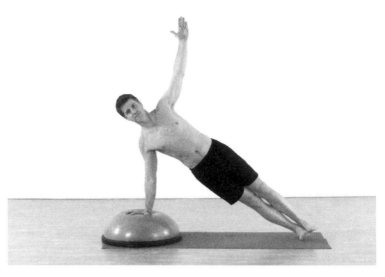

BALANCE TRAINING DEFINED

Balance training is often linked to stability training. You'll work your body in a position or a series of positions that occur during movement, while co-contractions of the muscles on either side of the joints help maintain that specific position. In other words, muscles on both sides of your joint assist in stabilization. In real life, your body needs a variety of muscles to keep you steady on your feet and to help move you as well.

it's not an unavoidable consequence of aging. Regardless of your age, you can be thrown off balance by a puddle of water or uneven pavement. Falls occur any time, any place, in any situation, from getting out of a bathtub to skiing a black diamond slope. You are not immune from falling. You can, however, take simple steps to improve your balance and reduce your risk of falling. That's where these workouts come in. These stability workouts provide both strength and balance challenges in an integrated manner. Balance is just like muscle strength—if you don't use it, you lose it.

Balance Benefits

In a healthy body *regardless of your age*, you will turn on and tone up just about every muscle in your body and improve

your overall quality of movement with these stability exercises. You or your body will never get bored because these exercises will constantly keep you on your toes, and as long as your muscles don't get bored, your body will change.

These workouts have many other benefits, the least of which is a Wow! Body:

• You'll hone your mindful training skills, simultaneously training your balance reaction. As you train, your mind and muscles become more synchronized. As a result, you can stand on one leg or catch yourself from a disastrous fall without even thinking about it. Remember, stability and strength play critical roles in all physical movements.

• You'll strengthen your core muscles. By focusing on your center, you'll strengthen the stabilizing muscles of your trunk. A strong core will reduce strain on your limbs and keep the injury-prone areas, such as your lower back, healthy.

• You'll improve your posture. Good posture requires strength. By strengthening the deep stabilizing muscles of your torso, you'll build a strong foundation for your spinal bones and have plenty of strength to hold your shoulders high and keep your joints in place. Good posture also translates into less injury and a healthier body—you'll look better, too!

• You'll enhance your neuromuscular function. By training your balance and muscles, you'll sharpen your nervous system. Skeletal muscle will not contract unless it receives a signal from your nervous system. Since balance is the foundation for all human movement, you'll keep your neuromuscular system functioning at an optimal level, too.

• You'll fine-tune your sensory systems. By simultaneously working on balance and strength moves, you'll sharpen your neuromuscular reaction, which will increase movement efficiency regardless of the activity.

• You'll decrease your chances of an injury. When your body is strong and stable, your daily performance will improve, as will your body confidence.

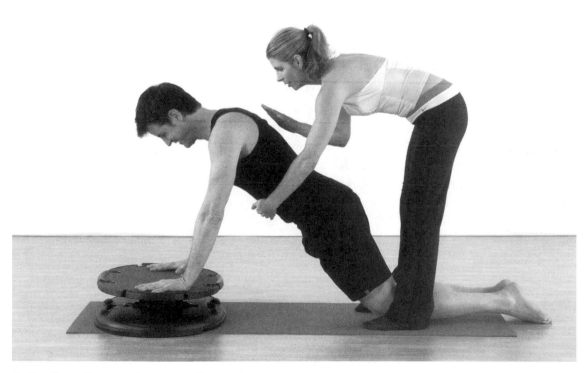

Author Karon Karter makes some adjustments.

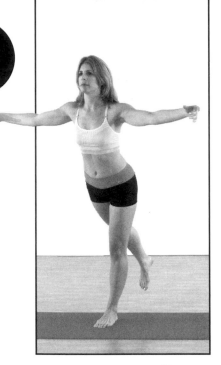

where's my body?

The ability to balance is a complex process that depends on three major components: 1) Sensory systems must first figure out where your body is in space; 2) your brain processes that information, makes essential changes, and directs those changes; and 3) your muscles and joints receive that information to keep you steady on your feet.

Sensory systems are continually trying to figure out where your body's position is in space by processing information in the brain and asking your muscles and joints to coordinate movements so you can balance. These systems include your eyes, inner ears, feet, ankles, and joints. Your eyes collect data and tell you if the environment around you is moving or still. Balance organs in your inner ears send messages as to whether you're upright, leaning, standing still, or moving. Pressure sensors on the bottom of your feet report which way is "up" by

the way you stand, and recognize whether the surface you're standing on is uneven or moving. With all this sensory input, your brain can accurately figure out where your body is in space, which way it's moving, and how quickly.

Let's say you kick your leg too high for optimal balance. To make corrections, your brain adds up all sensory input and in a blaze compares it to an internal blueprint of stored sensations. It then takes action. Your brain and spinal cord make last-minute adjustments by sending nerve

signals to dozens of muscles, instructing them to contract or relax as needed. Your brain compares your actual position with an image that it has learned somewhere along the way. This programmed internal blueprint, or muscle memory, is another component of sensory input and is called proprioception, meaning "own reception."

Proprioception is a sixth sense telling you how to react quickly in any moment in your life. You can, for example, balance on a snowboard for the first time or instinctively react within a

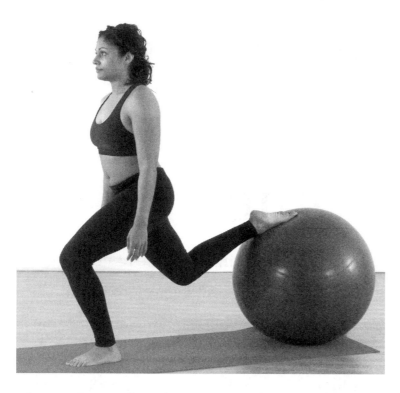

front of you. Then move slowly and consciously, not turning your head too quickly or else you might throw off your inner ear balance. Think about every subtle movement so you don't wobble—this is where mind and body unite. Finally, your head will remain stable and in line with your shoulders as your shoulders line up over your hips to maintain optimal or neutral spinal alignment. Specifically, your torso muscles will act as an anchor and stable point for your entire body. Think about it. Balance control takes a combination of many bodily systems; it will help if you begin to think in terms of eyes, ears, and core.

So it's true—your mind controls your muscles. *Balance Training* workouts create smart, strong muscles because your body will remember what you teach it, which is why it's so important to incorporate balance, brain, and strength challenges that will help you move more efficiently and safely. All of these systems are interrelated and, when you train this way, you'll create balance in your body. When it's all over, you'll have sexy, strong, sculpted muscles in places you've never imagined.

split second to avoid a car accident. Balance exercises simultaneously train your brain, nerves, and muscles to create smart muscles in a neurological way. As you train, your central nervous system makes and stores internal blueprints of learned responses that your body will later recall when needed in your everyday life. More specifically, you'll train your body and brain to recall balance and strength in relation to your body position and the whereabouts of each body part in space within that moment. Everyone possesses some degree of body sense, but

you can hone this skill just like any other fitness element.

So how will this affect you? You'll notice that these workouts challenge your balance and your body in a variety of positions. To help you stay steady on your feet, you'll repeat these steps: 1) Find your focus through use of your eyes, 2) work in optimal spinal alignment (see "Bringing Balance Home," page 8), and 3) engage your core muscles, which play a major role in stability.

You'll first depend on your eyes to help you balance. Find a fixed spot on the wall in

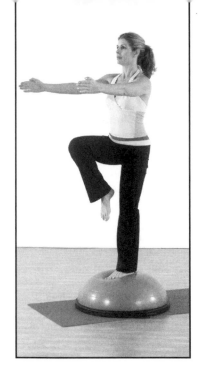

bringing balance home

It's time to get moving, but you're not sure where to begin. No problem! Here you'll learn how to align your body so you can work out safely. After that, all you'll need is a little space, a couple of easy-to-find props, and some good music to get you into the mood.

Balance in Your Body

Your muscles broadly fit into two categories: stabilizing, or postural, and movement. Stabilizing muscles stabilize your body while movement muscles move your body. More specifically, stabilizing muscles, such as your deep abdominal and back muscles, tend to be deep. Movement muscles, such as the quadriceps and hamstrings, are superficial, active, and often very tight from overuse.

These exercises strengthen a variety of muscles in your body while focusing on your torso muscles as a whole. Why? Because balance is linked to how strong your core muscles are. While there are many torso muscles, your deep ab and back muscles stabilize your spine (probably without you knowing it) in just about every position in your daily life—standing, kneeling, seated, side-lying, face down, and face up. If these muscles are weak, they tend to sag, making daily movements (including stability) difficult. In the end, weak postural muscles can't support your body. As a result, you might get a pot belly or have nagging twinges that may escalate into chronic pain. By focusing on your core muscles, you'll stabilize your spine so you can move safely and build strength within your torso muscles, specifically your deep postural muscles.

Core Competence

Your core muscles are made up of numerous muscles that overlap and extend from the base of your neck to the muscles between your legs. Because these muscles provide support for your torso plus stabilize your spine, it's critical that you strengthen them. Just about every daily movement you do requires core strength and stability.

Core stability depends on the strength of your core. To understand your musculature, imagine an onion and its many layers. You have four layers of abdominals, or abs. The most superficial layer is your *rectus abdominis*. You can literally see this muscle contract because it sits on the surface of your abdomen, attaching near your breastbone and ending near your pubic bone. Activate this muscle and you can bend forward or do a crunch. Peel away a layer and you'll find a network of oblique abdominals. The *internal and external obliques* crisscross your abdomen to assist in both stabilization and movement of your trunk. The external obliques are fairly shallow and are often visible if you have the six-pack ab look. They originate on the lower ribs and insert on the pelvis, while the internal obliques are much deeper, originating on the pelvis and inserting on the lower ribs. Between the two, they form an "X" across your center so that you can twist and bend at the waist. Peel away another layer and you'll find your deepest postural

abdominal, the *transversus abdominis*, or transverse. This abdominal muscle "wraps" around your trunk and lies directly against your spine; it stabilizes your spine by forming a deep girdle of support. When you strengthen this muscle, you reinforce your torso and help protect your lower back.

In every exercise, you'll focus on a deep exhalation to engage all of these ab muscles so that they can work together to create abdominal bracing, resulting in torso stability. There is growing evidence that your diaphragm is important to spinal stabilization because of that bracing feeling, or intra-abdominal pressure. When you perform these exercises correctly, you may feel a tightening around your waist as if a belt is cinching around it. You can also get this feeling by laughing or coughing—try it! Notice that your belly shrinks while it moves toward your spine.

Core muscles include your back muscles. They, too, assist in spinal stabilization (remember, two opposing muscle groups support a joint). Just like your front muscles, your back muscles are built upon layers. Most superficial are your *erector spinae*. This thick group of back muscles travels

the length of your spine, helping you bend your spine backward as in a back bend or a position called spinal extension. The *multifidus* is a lesser-known spinal stabilizing muscle that also travels the length of the spine. It spans three layers deep and is directly responsible for spinal stabilization.

A group of muscles, lying deep within the bottom of your pelvis, makes up your *pelvic floor*. These layered muscles provide hammock-like support from your pubic bone to your tailbone. Think of your pelvic floor as an elevator: when you're relaxed, your pelvic floor is at ground level; when engaged, it rises to the next floor. You can literally feel your pelvic floor lift, especially as you exhale, in the area between your belly button

FEET FIRST

Your foot is the foundation for standing, walking, running, and just about every balancing move you make in your daily life. You take nearly 10,000 steps each day, and your feet bear the weight of your body. Yet they seem to get the least amount of attention. When your feet are weak, so is your body. Clearly, healthy posture begins with a bare foot. In fact, poor foot alignment can contribute to needless aches and pains from the ground up—ankles, knees, hips, and back.

and pubic bone. All in all, your transverse, multifidus, diaphragm, and pelvic floor work in tandem to stabilize your spine, while the more superficial muscles support and move your spine. When fit and strong, these muscles come into action all on their own, which is why it's so important to focus on your core in each exercise. The strongest spine calls on many muscles, not just a few.

Total Body Stability: Neutral Spine

With every new student, I look for what I call "total body stability." In other words, I assess whether her hip and shoulder points are even and and still during all movement and whether she maintains a neutral spine as she exercises. This is my goal for you as well. To do this, let's go over two areas of your body: hip/pelvis and shoulder/scapula (shoulder blades). When aligned correctly, these complexes recruit muscles on both sides of the joint with equal

force to stabilize your shoulders, hips, and core—total body stability.

Neutral spine puts the least amount of stress on your body. In neutral spine, your joints, ligaments, tendons, muscles, and bones are properly aligned and will function as intended. In a perfect world, you would sit, stand, drive, and work out in a neutral spine position, but that is hardly the case. Sitting at your desk slumped over a computer or driving for hours hunched over the wheel can trigger the downward cycle of poor posture and muscle imbalances. Can't touch your toes? Inflexibility can also make it difficult to maintain neutral spine. If you don't focus on a neutral spine position, then you're reinforcing muscle imbalances in your body. Eventually, poor alignment can lead to permanently misaligned spinal bones and overwrought joints.

The good news is that body awareness is the first step, followed by strengthening your torso muscles, which both sta-

bilize and move your spine. Because your pelvis attaches to your spine and leg bones, its position directly plays a major role in lumbar or lower back stability. In fact, the position of your pelvis is often a good indication as to what is happening in the rest of the spine, so let's begin here.

Finding Neutral   To find a neutral position, lie on your back and bend your knees. Rest the palm of your hand on your pelvis, finding the point between the pubic bone and the bony point on your pelvis. Rest your fingers on your pubic bone while the palm of your hand lies flat on your hip bone. Tip your pubic bone to the ceiling, flattening your lower back to the floor (a position sometimes called *pelvic tilt*), so that your fingers lift toward the ceiling.

Yet if you tilt your pubic bone to the floor, creating a huge lower back arch (or anterior tilt position), the palm of your hand will rest high while your fingers lie low. This is an *anterior tilt*. In neutral pelvis,

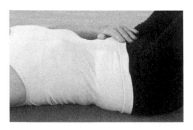

Neutral pelvis.

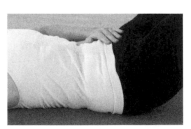

Pelvic tilt.

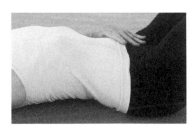

Anterior tilt.

the palm of your hand will rest flat and there's a slight arch in your lower back. Experiment with the pictures below. Move your pelvis back and forth (which is also a nice stretch), and then try to return to a neutral position.

Shoulder Stability Now notice the network of muscles and bones on your upper back. These muscles attach your shoulder blades, or the winged bones, to your back, keep you standing upright, help support movement of your arms, and stabilize your shoulder girdle. In each exercise, you'll keep your shoulders stable by stabilizing your shoulder blades because they directly influence the position of your shoulders.

Because your shoulders are dependent on your shoulder blades and the muscles that both move and stabilize them, you should have a basic understanding of the muscles involved. These muscles zigzag in different directions to perform many functions and to provide upper torso stability. For starters, a tiny stabilizing muscle called the *serratus anterior* wraps around your rib cage and helps your shoulder blades remain flat on your back. If your shoulder blades stick up or protrude, it may be because this muscle is weak. I

see this constantly in my classes: as students attempt to do a push-up, their shoulders lift to their ears while their shoulder blades stick out. Unfortunately, this misalignment can injure you, which is why it's so important to take it slow and build deep postural strength, as opposed to powering through an exercise to get it over with.

Working in harmony with your serratus is your *trapezius* muscle, which forms a big diamond on your back. The mid and lower traps help prevent your shoulders from lifting to your ears. Your *rhomboids*, which are located between your shoulder blades, also assist in keeping your shoulder blades flat on your back. The biggest muscle on your back, the *latissimus dorsi*, or lats, supports and stabilizes your shoulder blades, depending on the movement. On the opposite side of your upper spine lie your chest muscles, or *pectoralis*. They, too, assist in shoulder blade stabilization.

To understand how your shoulder blades move your shoulders, try moving your shoulder blades in these four positions:

Shoulder blade elevation: Lift your shoulders to your ears.

Shoulder blade depression, or *proper form:* Lower your shoul-

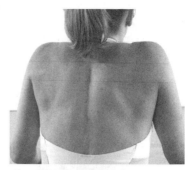
Shoulder blade elevation.

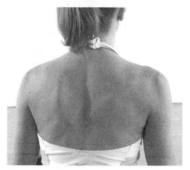
Shoulder blade depression, or proper form.

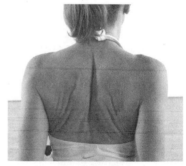
Shoulder blade protraction.

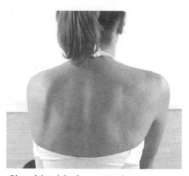
Shoulder blade retraction.

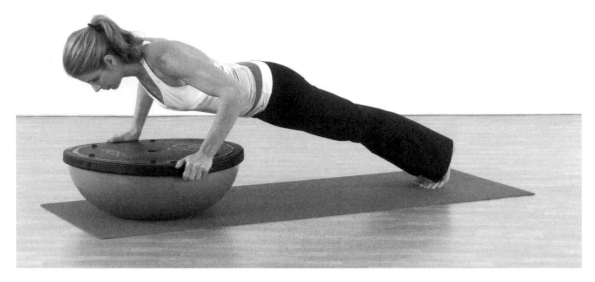

ders away from your ears so your shoulder blades slide down and lie flat on your back.

Shoulder blade protraction: Move your shoulder blades together. This position opens your chest, and you might feel a stretch across your chest as well.

Shoulder blade retraction: Move your shoulder blades away from each other. This position closes your chest and rounds your shoulders forward.

Ideally, your goal is to work with your shoulder blades flat on your back, sliding them down into place as shown on page 11. If any of these muscles are weak, imbalances can lead to poor shoulder alignment, tension in the neck, chest, or upper back, headaches, and chronic pain. So as you move from exercise to

exercise, keep your shoulders even and stable to build optimal upper back strength and good posture. However, sometimes maintaining shoulder stability isn't always easy. If you can't keep your shoulders in place, start the exercise over. Eventually, you'll gain awareness and strength.

Of course, as you progress, the main goal is to focus on the torso as a whole to maintain total body stability. Keep in mind that your body is only

as strong as the muscles that stabilize your frame as well as the muscles that move your body—all make up a carefully balanced system. If one set of muscles falls short, then eventually your entire body may feel the nagging aches and pains. Sadly, pain travels and has a way of haunting you. Your best defense is to exercise with proper alignment in the first place. These exercises will strengthen your muscles as an entire system, from inside and

BENEFITS OF A NEUTRAL SPINE

- Neutral spine helps you exercise safely. By exercising in a stable position, you'll train your muscles correctly from the beginning.
- Neutral spine enhances overall posture. As you know, strong stabilizing muscles help keep your spinal bones in place. Neutral position equals good posture, and you'll eventually learn to feel what bad posture feels like. As a result, you'll learn how to adjust poor alignment while you sit, stand, or walk, whether you're at work, home, or in an exercise class.
- Neutral spine decreases your risk of injury. If you continue to reinforce bad form, an occasional twinge may escalate into something worse, such as chronic pain.

out. Sure, your abs will look good in next year's swimsuit but it's your body that will feel good 20 years from now.

Hip and Foot Stabilization Standing stability exercises are a necessary first step because they work all the muscles in your legs while challenging your hip stability. Hip stabilization is the ability to keep your hips stable, meaning the two hip points on your pelvis are even as if you could draw a straight line from hip point to hip point. Two primary muscles lie deep within the

hip area: the *gluteus medius* and *gluteus minimus*. Your gluteus medius connects to the outer rim of your pelvis to the upper thighbone and runs down the side of your leg, whereas the gluteus minimus lies much deeper underneath the medius. The *gluteus maximus* is your butt muscle; it's the most superficial of this group and can also help in keeping your hips stable.

Of course, to create stability within your hips, you need to look at the opposite muscle group—your inner thighs.

Collectively, these muscles are *adductors*, and they move your legs toward your body. *Abductors*, the muscles on the side of your thighs, move your legs away from your body. These muscles, in conjunction with your core muscles, help stabilize the lower half of your body: your hips and pelvis.

As for your lower leg muscles, the *tibialis anterior* is located on the outer front shin and the *peroneus longus* and *brevis* are on the outer calf. These help keep you steady on your feet.

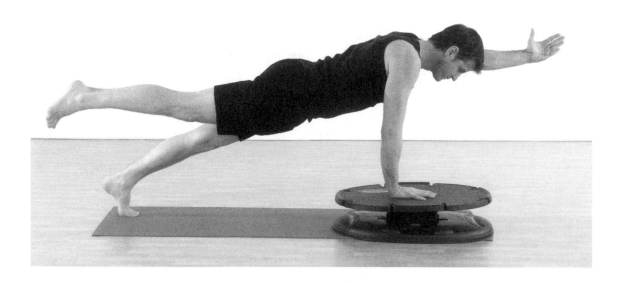

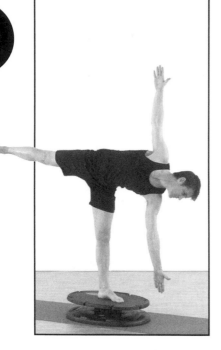

tips for a safer workout

As with any fitness program, you risk getting injured. Keep in mind that stability props increase the intensity of any exercise, so please use your best judgment and try not to advance yourself too quickly. Regardless if you're a fitness buff or a first-timer, focus on good form and self-control. The good news is if you fall, you're not too far from the ground! Below are a few precautions:

Get a medical checkup or consult your physician before starting any fitness program, especially if your doctor has said that you have a heart condition.

If you have balance issues or have any dizziness, don't proceed before talking to your doctor.

If you experience any pain, especially in your chest, while exercising, stop immediately.

Pay attention to your form. Maintain a neutral spine position because it's important to the overall integrity of your body and each exercise.

Remove obstacles, such as papers and clothing, and anything that may interfere with your balance workout from your workout area.

Keep your workout area well lit.

Exercise in a big area so you won't roll into a sharp object such as the edge of a coffee table.

Invest in a not-too-soft non-slip mat and use it for the ball, BOSU, and balance board workouts. These props are farther from the ground so a softer surface can help break your fall.

Don't exercise on a slippery surface.

Exercise with bare feet to increase your sensory feedback and stability.

Notice that you'll get a variety of tips with each exercise. Use them; they provide good cues to help you do the exercise correctly.

Don't jerk or swing your body into position. Stabilize

your spine and use muscle, not momentum.

Move thoughtfully and slowly to feel the exercises in your body. Take your time and exercise at your level of fitness. The exercises in this book are divided into beginner, intermediate, and advanced and are meant to progress from easy to most difficult; it's okay to take your time before advancing. If you advance too soon, you may get hurt. Training incorrectly or with improper body alignment will only set you back emotionally and physically.

Warm up with a cardio workout, such as walking, running, swimming, or bicycling, before these workouts. Don't blow off your warm-up! Muscles need to warm up gradually in order to not send them into muscle shock, which could cause injury.

Your muscles need to cool down, too. Take a few minutes to stretch each major muscle group.

Drink lots of water. If you're thirsty, it's too late.

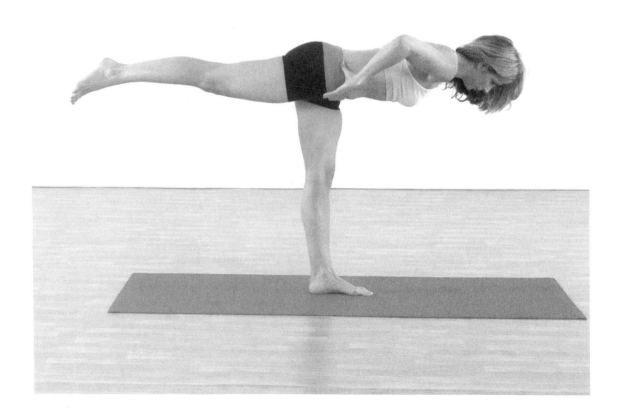

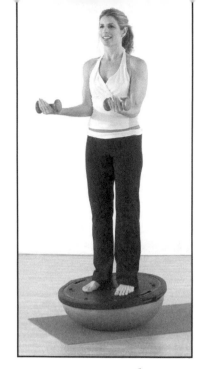

what you need: props

There are many types of equipment to choose from and you don't have to purchase every piece of equipment shown below. These props are interchangeable and work for some of the same exercises from workout to workout. I do, however, recommend buying a foam roller because it's cheap and versatile. Later on, you can purchase a more expensive prop so you can continue to challenge your muscles. If you have a gym membership, you can work with a personal trainer to get the most out of this book.

Because stability exercises are advanced in general, most of you will fall under the category of beginner unless you've been training on a specific prop. Keep in mind that not all of you will respond to the same exercises and props. That's why *Balance Training* has over 60 exercises featuring a variety of props as well as variations or modifications. Choose what's best for you. The most important thing is that you work with good

form! Pay attention to how you're holding your body in each exercise. Remember, your goal is total body stability so don't forget to reiterate the total body stability principles.

If you're doing an exercise on a certain prop and find that it's too hard, try doing that exact exercise on the floor without the prop yet maintain proper alignment. If a student of mine has never trained on a stability prop, I'll first teach proper alignment without

props. If she can maintain good form, then I'll add more challenging versions with props.

Below is a brief list of the props used in this book.

Foam Roller

Foam rollers come in a variety of sizes, lengths, textures, and materials. Good for students of all levels, they're relatively inexpensive and are ideal for increasing core strength while giving your spine support. What you'll see in the "Foam

Roller Workout" is a standard three-foot-long, six-inch-diameter foam roller; it runs about $18–$20.

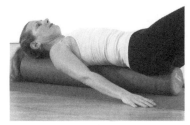

Foam roller.

Balance Cushion

Balance cushions also come in all sizes, colors, and materials. These are wonderful training tools because they're low to the ground in case you fall; some balance cushions are textured and can help you from slipping off—great for beginners. The one used in this book is a standard cushion, about 13½" diameter x 3"

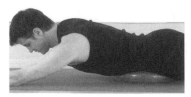

Balance cushion.

high. Average price ranges from $20–$30.

BOSU Balance Trainer

The BOSU is an air-filled dome that means "both sides utilized," meaning you can train on either side. The BOSU challenges your stability and strength in just about every body position. You can kneel, sit, lie, stand, and walk on the BOSU to enhance your balance skills. A standard BOSU is about 26" diameter x 10" high and weighs 15 pounds; the one pictured runs about $120.

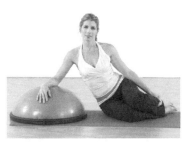

BOSU.

Balance Board

Balance boards pivot on an axis, moving in all planes of movement to challenge your strength and stability—great for more-advanced students. As with the BOSU, a variety of exercises can be done on them in a number of positions. Balance boards tend to be the most challenging piece of equipment, so be careful. Balance boards, too, come in different sizes and shapes. I

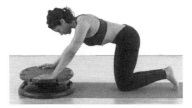

Balance board.

use the Reebok Core Board, priced from $130–$150.

Balance Ball

Balance balls are available in a variety of colors, sizes, and qualities. The ball is a versatile and inexpensive prop, but very challenging for most beginners because it's very unstable and higher off the ground. Beginners—you may want to start on the foam roller. Most women use a medium-sized ball (55cm). However, to make sure you have the right-sized ball for your height, sit on the ball and check that your knees fall even with or slightly above your hips. When you're ready to purchase a ball, consider choosing an anti-burst ball for your protection.

Once you're done reviewing this important introductory material, turn to Part 2 and choose your workout—it's time to get moving and bring balance home. Good luck!

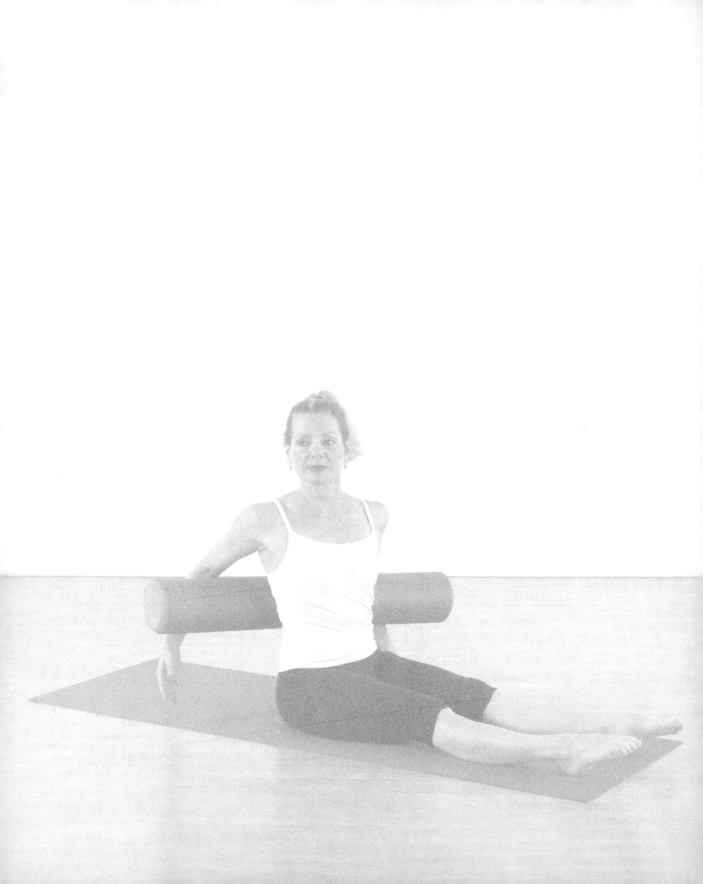

part two:
the workouts

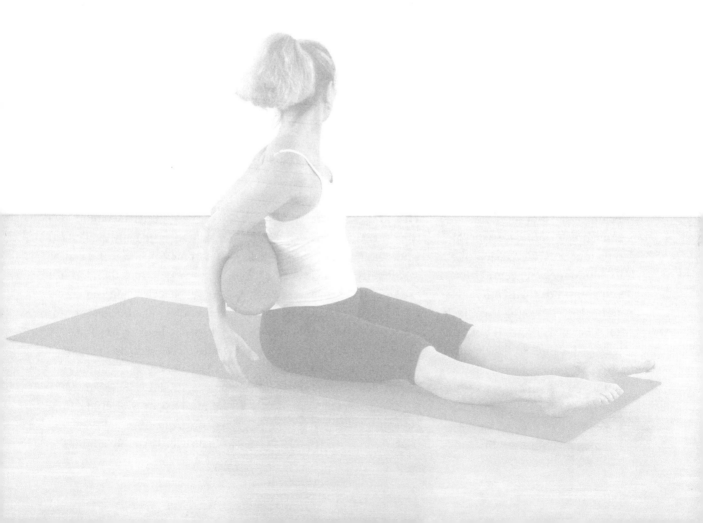

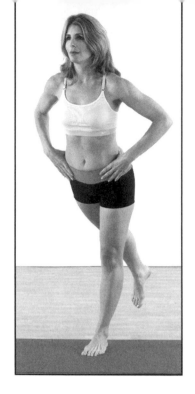

workouts overview

The *Balance Training* workouts in this section are a fun and effective addition to your weekly fitness routine. They also easily allow you to incorporate the important elements of cross-training. You can do these workouts for months because each workout increases in strength and stability challenges, progressing from beginner to advanced. Total time for each workout is 45 to 60 minutes.

On Monday, you might do a quick 15-minute cardio warm-up and follow it up with the One-Legged Workout; on Wednesday, you could do the Foam Roller Workout after some quick cardio. Or you can do a longer cardio session of 30 to 40 minutes and round off your fitness day with strength and balance by using the Quick Total Body Workout. If you're pressed for time and can't make it to the gym, feel free to do one of these workouts instead of your strength training for that day—just try to warm up with five minutes of cardio first. In the end, you'll still be strengthening your body, but you'll also be including a balance challenge.

The Progression

Note that the exercises in each workout are organized in order of difficulty, from easy to extreme. The first four workouts also appear in this order so that the One-Legged Workout is the simplest and the Extreme Prop Workout the hardest. To get the best results, start with the first workout to build the strength you'll need for the rest of the workouts. How can you tell when you're ready to advance to the next workout? When you're stable on your feet and can maintain proper spinal form.

These exercises should keep you and your body challenged for some time. If at the end of the year you find that you need more exercises, you can combine workouts, but just try to work the body as a whole—hips, core, and shoulders. Remember, you're building strength and stability to improve your overall life performance. A total body makeover is simply a bonus.

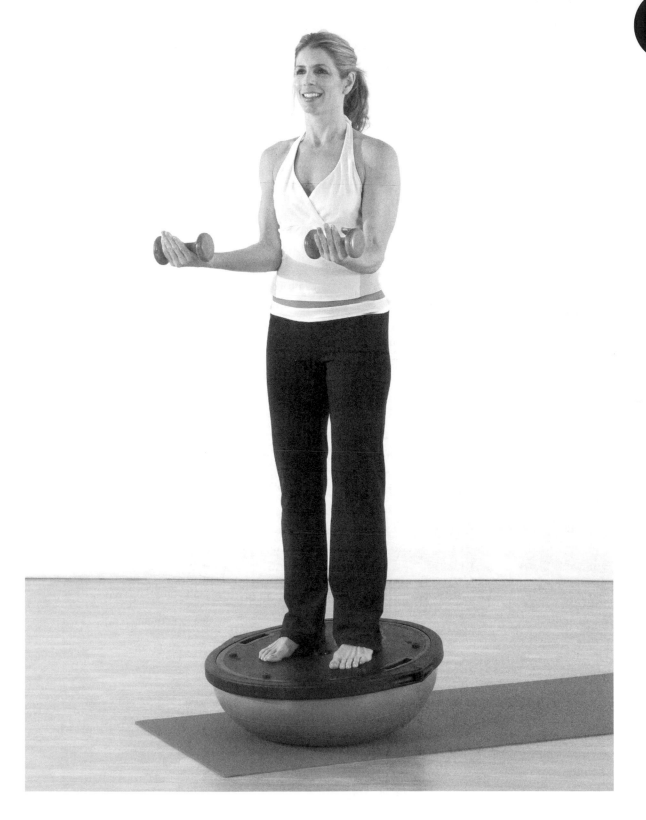

Workout 1: Get a Leg Up
The One-Legged Workout

Imagine slender legs, a lifted butt, and smoking-hot abs—this lower body workout will sculpt your bottom half sexy and leave you looking amazing from head to toe. In this one-legged workout, you'll generate force from the ground up and strengthen the muscles in your feet, legs, and hips while challenging your core stability. A great starting place for all levels. *Do this sequence for three to four weeks to develop enough strength before using the stability props.*

In this workout, you'll work your leg in just about every angle to challenge a variety of muscles while focusing on hip and core stability. As you move in and out of these exercises, your center of gravity will shift from side to side over your foot. This delicate dance—inner to outer foot, outer to inner foot—will continue while you're trying to keep your balance in check. The primary muscles involved are the *tibialis anterior*, located on outer front shin, and the *peroneus longus* and *brevis* on the outer calf. Although these muscles are small, they're heavy hitters in foot and ankle stabilization, and will strengthen as time goes on.

How do you know? You will waver less as your foot makes fewer muscular corrections.

Safe Start

As you move from one exercise to exercise, don't stop. Complete the entire routine on one leg and then switch legs to complete the same exercises on the other leg. Keep in mind that balancing on one leg can be extremely challenging and frustrating, especially because your other leg is moving, compromising your stability that much more. So keep it slow at first by beginning with the first three exercises: One-Legged Front Kick, One-Legged Side Kick, and One-Legged Side Passé. After you feel grounded, add three more exercises and so forth. Since this workout is your first introduction to stability training, let's go over a few tips that are specific to this workout.

- Gaze on a spot on the wall and don't look anywhere else during this routine.
- Focus on your breathing, especially your exhale, to engage your core muscles to help keep you steady.
- Maintain good foot alignment

by pressing firmly down on the three corners of your foot into the floor: center of your heel, big-toe joint, and pinky-toe joint.

- Align your upper body over your hips, and engage core muscles to help keep you from wobbling as your leg moves.
- Watch for sloppiness—as the moves increase in difficulty, your body might sacrifice good form for bad form: sinking into your waist, hunching your shoulders, turning out the working hip, twisting your torso, or just working the leg incorrectly. Sloppiness usually means fatigue; it's okay to stop and then regroup with good alignment.
- Begin with your weaker leg first.
- If you have trouble balancing, use the wall for support or hold your hands out to your sides like a tightrope walker.

ONE-LEGGED WORKOUT: EXERCISES

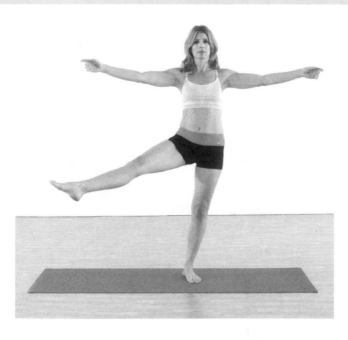

Workout 2: On a Roll
The Foam Roller Workout

This workout focuses on deepening your connection with your core muscles and challenges your spine in all of its natural movements (flexion, extension, and rotation). You'll learn how to engage your core muscles while holding your body balanced on a foam roller, strengthening your core for the more advanced work to come. This workout is outstanding for students of all levels because not only is the round tube close to the ground (just in case you fall), its comfortable surface provides postural support, especially for your spine and neck. After mastering this workout, you should have a good amount of core strength that will allow you to move on to more challenging props.

Stability Tips

• This workout increases in intensity as it progresses. For example, bent knees make the exercise easier whereas straight legs increase the workload of your core stabilizers. Likewise, moving legs and arms are the most challenging.

• Keep your legs and arms close to your core to make the exercise easier. As the legs and arms move farther and farther away, the intensity increases.

• If you get tired, rest. Less is always better if good form is practiced.

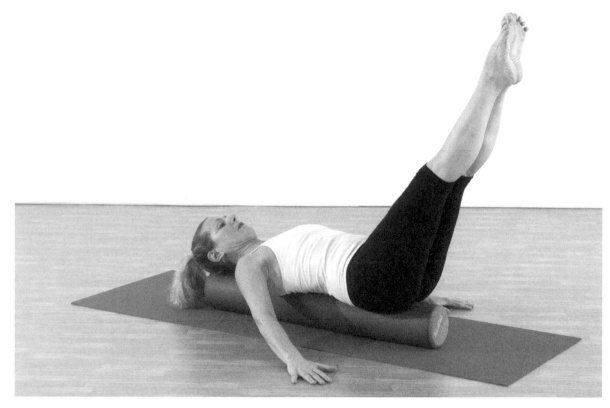

ROLLER WORKOUT: EXERCISES

Workout 3: Roll Off the Jiggle
The Ball Workout

Are you ready to rock and roll? This workout focuses on total body stability while building strength in your entire body. Because the ball wobbles, the exercises are more demanding.

Ball workouts tend to turn up the heat for your core and increase the balance challenge. The balancing act is worth it because you'll intensify the workload for your muscles,

engaging just about every muscle in your body. Translation: mega calories burned—think "roll off the jiggle"! Take your time—and remember to work with good form. Have fun!

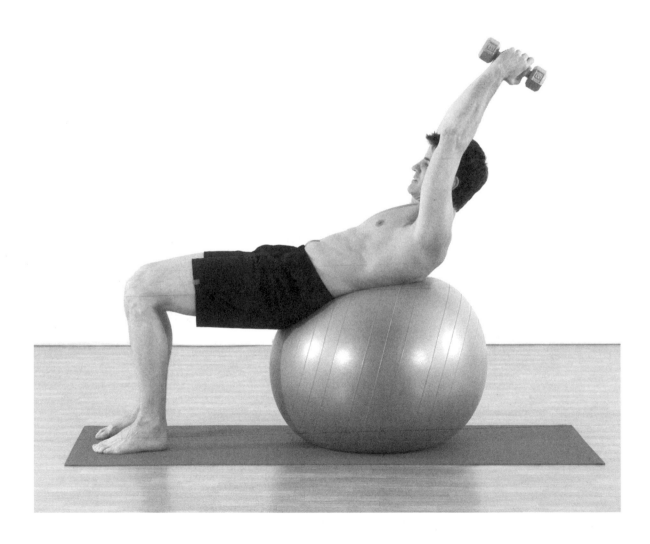

BALL WORKOUT: EXERCISES

Workout 4: Your Balanced and Best Body
The Multi-Prop Workout

This workout blends total body stability challenges with total body strengthening moves to engage all of your muscles as well as your balance. Much of what you'll do is integrate various muscle groups in a variety of positions on all kinds of stability props, challenging your body in extreme ways. You'll also see modifications, but this workout should only be done after months of building your total body stability. You can use any prop you'd like, and remember that good form is vital to building a balanced body with lots of strength, stability, and, of course, "Wow!" results.

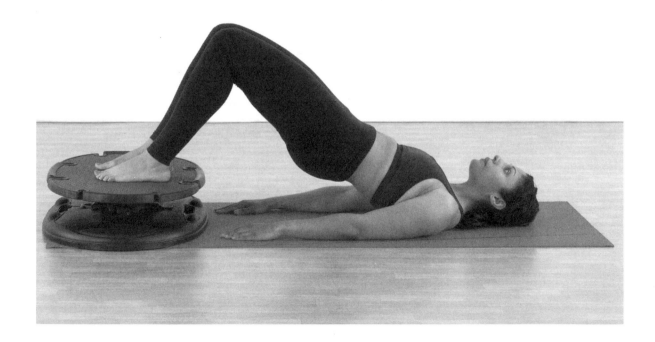

MULTI-PROP WORKOUT: EXERCISES

Workout 5: Five Total Body Exercises
The Quick Total Body Workout

Even if you don't have as much time to exercise as you'd like, you can still maintain and improve your balance and strength. This quick, full-body workout is available in three levels of difficulty and takes a total of 10 minutes to do. Just remember to do at least five minutes of cardio beforehand to get the best results.

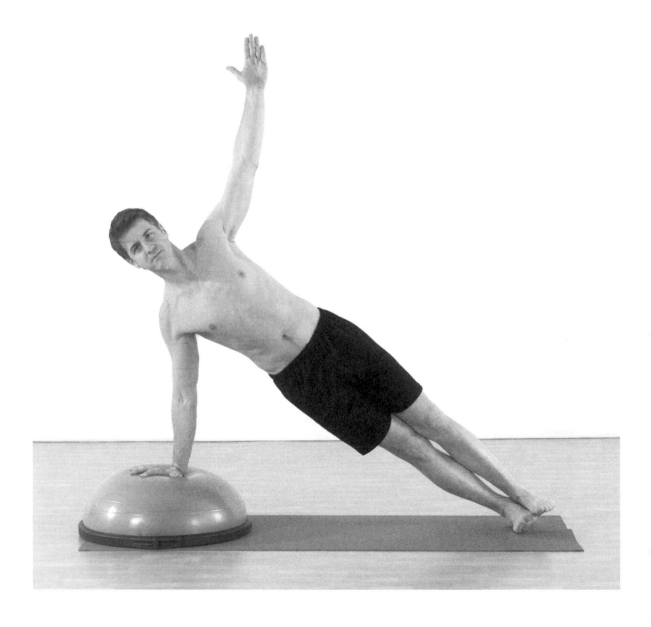

QUICK TOTAL BODY WORKOUT: EXERCISES

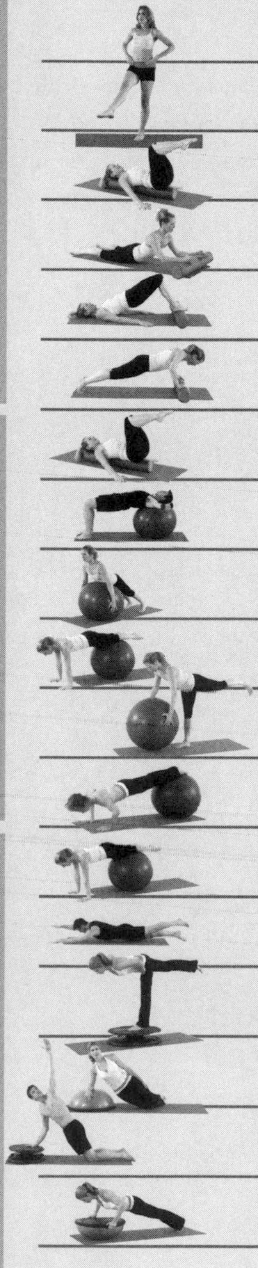

beginner

	PAGE	EXERCISE
	38	One-Legged Front Kick
	52	Bent Knees on Roller
	60	Spinal Extension on Roller
	61	Shoulder Bridge on Roller
	64	Push-Up on Roller

intermediate

	52	Bent Knees on Roller
	68	Ball Bridge with Arm Circles (add weights)
	72	Spinal Extension on Ball
	78	Plank on Ball
	75	One-Legged Deadlift with Ball
	84	*Bonus:* Ball Pike and Push-Up Combination

advanced to extreme

	78	Plank on Ball
	91	Spinal Cross-Extension on Balance Cushion (Swimming)
	103	One-Legged Deadlift on Balance Board
	94	Side Plank on BOSU
	97	Plank Twist on Balance Board
	98	*Bonus:* Push-Up on BOSU

Workout 6: The Best Total Body Workout

This workout involves a combination of all the workouts to mix things up a little. Notice that each workout combines strengthening your hips, core, and shoulders while moving you from standing to sitting. Why? To burn more calories and mega fat, and build more muscles. You'll tone your body from head to toe—and all those muscles you never knew you had.

TOTAL BODY WORKOUT: EXERCISES

beginner

	PAGE	EXERCISE
	36	Foot Strengthener
	38	One-Legged Front Kick
	42	One-Legged Parallel Leg Lift
	43	One-Legged Back Leg Lift
	50	Moving Arms on Roller
	52	Bent Knees on Roller
	54	Toe Dips on Roller
	59	Seated Spinal Twist with Roller
	87	Cat on Balance Board
	90	Spinal Extension on Balance Cushion
	78	Beginner Plank on Ball
	100	One-Legged Stand on BOSU (or balance cushion)
	86	Drape Over Ball

intermediate

advanced to extreme

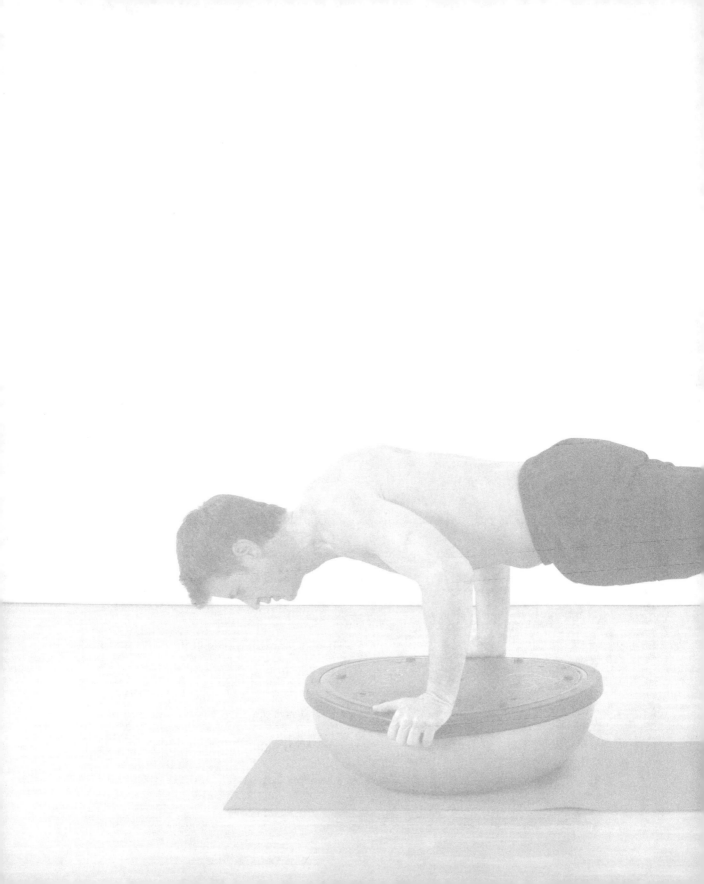

part three:
the
exercises

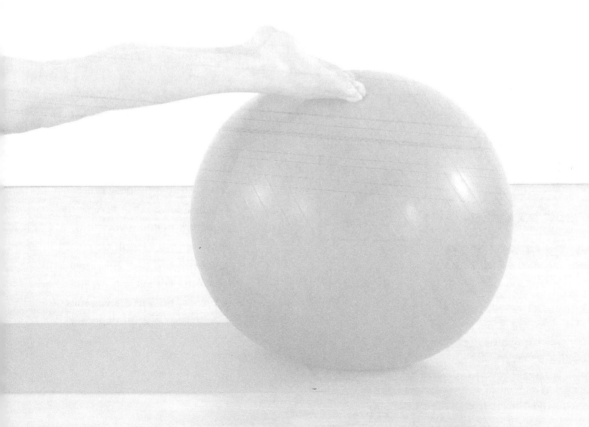

foot strengthener

Benefits: Strengthens the muscles, ligaments, and tendons of your foot

STARTING POSITION: Lie on your back and wrap an elastic band lengthwise around your foot, from your toes to your heel. While holding the band, straighten your leg. Keep your foot in a neutral position, and apply slight, even pressure to the three corners of your foot: heel, big toe, and little toe. Breathe normally throughout the exercise.

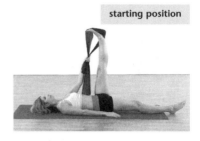
starting position

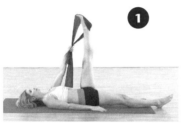
1

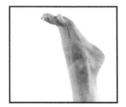

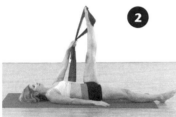
2

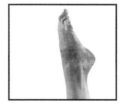

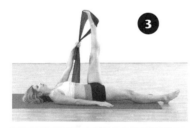
3

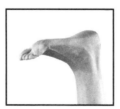

1 Point the heel of your foot, yet keep your toes relaxed. Your foot is in a half-point position.

2 Point your toes so that your entire foot is in a point position.

3 Keeping your foot pointed, flex your toes back toward your face.

Return to starting position. Repeat 5 times, then reverse the sequence, pointing your toes, pointing your heel, flexing just your toes, and then flexing your foot. After completing the full sequence, do 5 to 8 ankle rolls. Repeat sequence on the other leg.

TIPS

- Maintain proper foot alignment so you don't strengthen your muscles incorrectly.
- Take your time to fully stretch and strengthen your foot.
- If your foot cramps, rest for a second. Don't give up—as your muscles strengthen, your foot will stop cramping.

Benefits: Strengthens the stabilizing muscles of your hips and core while tightening and toning your leg muscles

This exercise will help you determine how stable you are in general. Notice your ankle shifting from side to side.

STARTING POSITION: Stand with your heels together and straighten your arms by your sides. Make sure your hip points face forward and remain even in order to build core and hip stability. Engage your abs from navel to spine. Lift from the top of your head, tuck your chin, and drop your shoulders. Keep your knees active but not hyperextended or locked, and align them between your second and third toes.

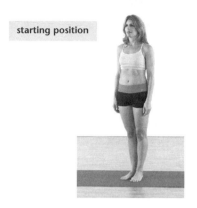

starting position

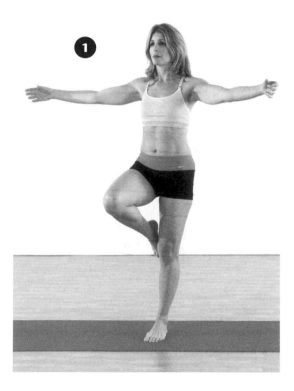

1 Bend and raise your knee until your foot lifts to the midline of your body. Try to lift your knee to hip height. Breathe normally but focus on the exhale to pull your belly button to your spine.

Complete 5 breath cycles, inhaling for 3 counts and exhaling deeply for 5 counts, then lower your foot back to starting position. Repeat on the opposite leg.

Eventually, you will increase the count to 5 inhalations and 8 exhalations.

TIPS
- On every exhale, try to feel the bracing of your torso to engage your core muscles.
- If standing on one leg is too difficult, then work near a wall.

ADVANCED: Try this exercise with your eyes closed.

one-legged front kick

Benefits: Strengthens the stabilizing muscles of your hips and core while tightening and toning your leg muscles

STARTING POSITION: Stand with your heels together and your arms along your sides. Your hip points face forward and remain even. Engage your abs from navel to spine. Lift from the top of your head, tuck your chin, and drop your shoulders. Keep your knees active but not hyperextended or locked, and align them between your second and third toes.

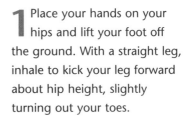

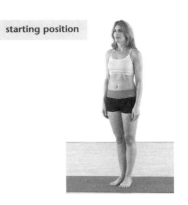

starting position

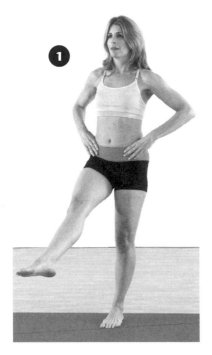

1 Place your hands on your hips and lift your foot off the ground. With a straight leg, inhale to kick your leg forward about hip height, slightly turning out your toes.

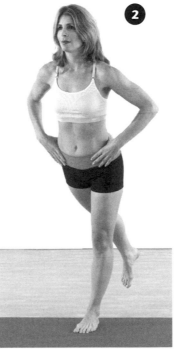

2 Exhale to kick your leg back behind you, engaging your buttocks. Your leg is moving from front to back as if you're sweeping the floor with your foot. Make sure your back does not arch as your leg swings back.

Repeat 5 to 8 times then switch sides.

ADVANCED: To increase the intensity, you can add a small kick as you kick front and back. The rhythm is kick, small kick.

one-legged side kick

Benefits: Strengthens the stabilizing muscles of your hips and core while tightening and toning your leg muscles

STARTING POSITION: Stand with your heels together and raise your arms to shoulder height. Your hip points face forward and remain even. Engage your abs from navel to spine. Lift from the top of your head, tuck your chin, and drop your shoulders. Keep your knees active but not hyperextended or locked, and align them between your second and third toes.

starting position

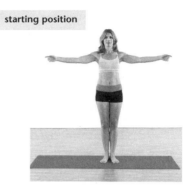

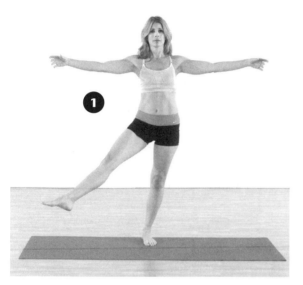

1 Inhale to lift your leg to the side, letting your knee lead the way.

2 Exhale to lower your raised heel to your standing heel, activating your inner thigh muscles.

Repeat 5 to 8 times then switch sides.

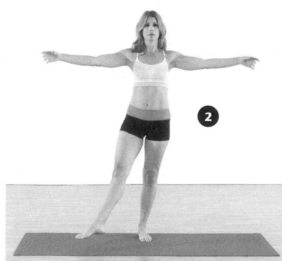

ADVANCED: Add a couple of quick heel beats next to the standing leg's heel; it's a small kick-kick so the heel of the moving leg touches the heel of the standing leg. You can also increase the workload by adding self-resistance as you lower your leg.

one-legged side passé

Benefits: Strengthens the stabilizing muscles of your hips and core while tightening and toning your leg muscles

STARTING POSITION: Stand with your heels together and raise your arms to shoulder height. Your hip points face forward and remain even. Engage your abs from navel to spine. Lift from the top of your head, tuck your chin, and drop your shoulders. Keep your knees active but not hyperextended or locked, and align them between your second and third toes.

starting position

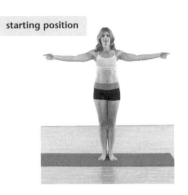

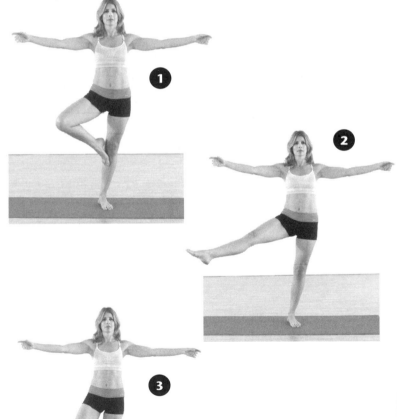

1 Inhale to open your hip so your knee turns to the side, revealing your inner thigh. Bend your knee and slide your heel along the inside of your inner thigh.

2 Continue to inhale as you straighten your leg to the side.

3 Exhale to lower your leg to the floor, leading with your heel to engage your inner thigh muscles.

Repeat 5 to 8 times, and then reverse the direction of the side passé. Switch sides.

TIPS

• Try to keep your knee open to the side to stretch your hip.
• If you lose your balance, don't lift your leg as high. Start small and then increase the range of motion.

one-legged leg circle

Benefits: Strengthens the stabilizing muscles of your hips and core while tightening and toning your leg muscles

STARTING POSITION: Stand with your heels together and your arms along your sides. Your hip points face forward and remain even. Engage your abs from navel to spine. Lift from the top of your head, tuck your chin, and drop your shoulders. Keep your knees active but not hyperextended or locked, and align them between your second and third toes.

starting position

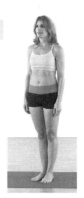

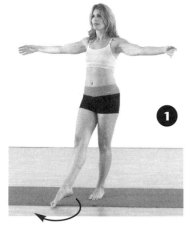

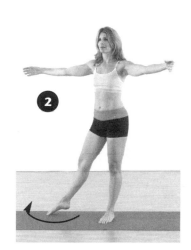

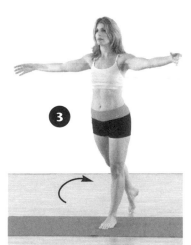

1 Inhale and raise your arms to shoulder height as you lift your leg to the side, just about an inch.

2–3 Exhale and, leading from your hip, circle your leg. Keep your circles small so that your inner thighs touch one another with every circle. Your heel will slightly touch the heel of the standing leg.

Circle your leg 5 to 8 times and then reverse direction. Switch sides.

TIPS

• Move from your inner thighs—this results in slim and trim legs.

one-legged parallel leg lift

Benefits: Strengthens the stabilizing muscles of your hips and core while tightening and toning your leg muscles

STARTING POSITION: Stand with your toes parallel and raise your arms to shoulder height. Your hip points face forward and remain even. Engage your abs from navel to spine. Lift from the top of your head, tuck your chin, and drop your shoulders. Keep your knees active but not hyperextended or locked, and align them between your second and third toes.

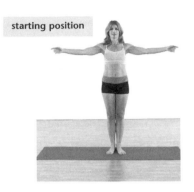

starting position

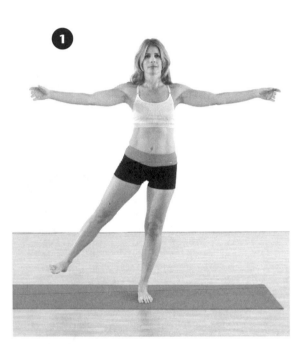

1

1 Inhale to lift your right leg to the side. Keep your leg parallel to engage your gluteus medius.

2 Exhale and, squeezing your inner thighs, slowly lower your leg.

Repeat 5 to 8 times then switch sides.

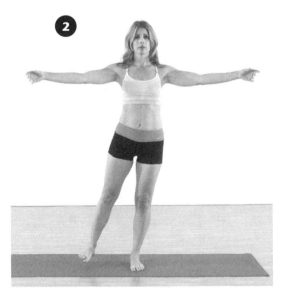

2

Benefits: Strengthens the stabilizing muscles of your hips and core while tightening and toning your leg muscles

STARTING POSITION: Stand with your toes parallel and raise your arms to shoulder height. Lean forward slightly so your hip points point toward the floor; keep them even and stable. Engage your abs, lifting your belly button toward your spine to strengthen your core muscles, especially as you lean forward. Lift from the top of your head, tuck your chin, and drop your shoulders. Keep your knees active but not hyperextended or locked, and align them between your second and third toes.

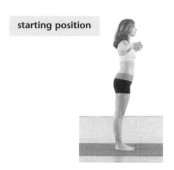

starting position

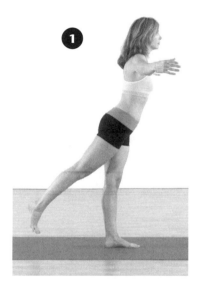

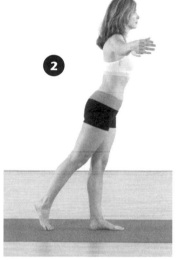

1 Inhale to lift your leg to the back, leading with your heel to engage your buttocks muscle. Nothing moves but your leg!

2 Exhale to lower your leg to the starting position.

Repeat 5 to 8 times then switch sides.

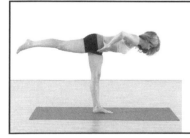

ADVANCED: Lift your leg as high as you can while your torso lowers to the floor. Ideally, your head, torso, and leg are in a straight line. This exercise will turn on major hamstring muscles on the standing leg, plus you'll see it later as a one-legged deadlift (pages 75 and 103) on a variety of props.

one-legged bicycle

Benefits: Strengthens the stabilizing muscles of your hips and core while tightening and toning your leg muscles

STARTING POSITION: Stand with your toes parallel and your arms along your sides. Your hip points face forward and remain even. Engage your abs from navel to spine. Lift from the top of your head, tuck your chin, and drop your shoulders. Keep your knees active but not hyperextended or locked, and align them between your second and third toes.

starting position

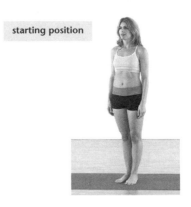

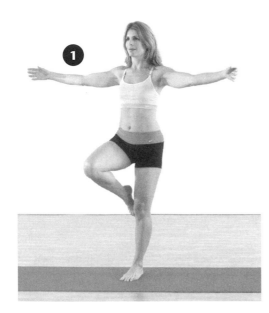

1 Inhale to raise your arms to shoulder height as you bend your knee and lift it to the ceiling. Focus on your core stability to keep your body still while the leg works.

2 Exhale as you straighten your leg, flexing your foot.

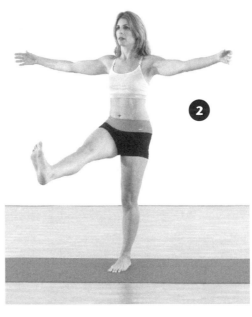

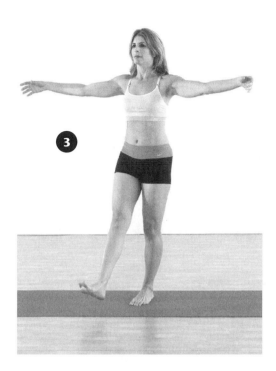

3–4 Continue to exhale as you lower the straight leg to the floor and then behind you, engaging your hamstrings.

Repeat 5 to 8 times and then reverse directions. Switch sides.

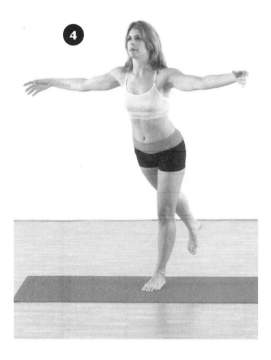

ADVANCED: To increase the intensity and turn on more hamstrings, drag your heel across the floor.

one-legged front leg kick

Benefits: Strengthens the stabilizing muscles of your hips and core while tightening and toning your leg muscles

STARTING POSITION: Stand with your toes parallel and raise your arms to shoulder height. Your hip points face forward and remain even. Engage your abs from navel to spine. Lift from the top of your head, tuck your chin, and drop your shoulders. Keep your knees active but not hyperextended or locked, and align them between your second and third toes.

starting position

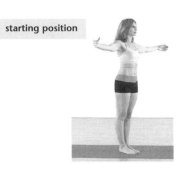

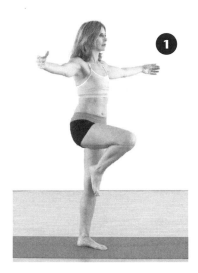

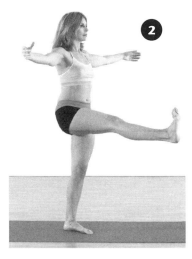

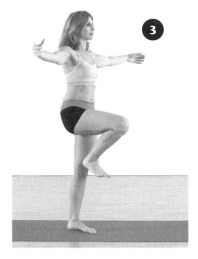

1 Lift your knee to hip height.

2 Inhale to slowly kick your leg until it's straight, engaging your quadriceps.

3 Exhale to bend your knee.

Repeat 5 to 8 times, and then switch legs.

TIPS

• Don't haphazardly kick your leg. Use self-control to engage as many muscles as possible.

one-legged back lunge

Benefits: Strengthens the stabilizing muscles of your hips and core while tightening and toning your leg muscles

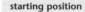

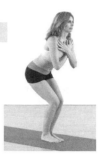

STARTING POSITION: From standing, bend your knees and slightly lean forward. Cross your wrists and place your hands near your chest.

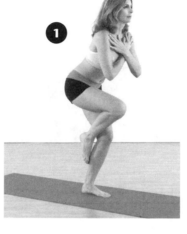

1 Lift your right knee toward your chest.

2 Inhale to slowly kick your right leg behind you as your left leg bends into a lunge position.

3 Exhale to return your right foot to starting position, slightly tapping your foot to the ground for balance. Maintain a lunge position as the right leg moves back and forth.

Repeat 5 to 8 kicks and then switch sides.

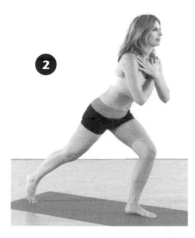

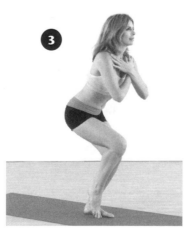

TIPS

- Keep your kicks small at first.
- The majority of your body weight is in your lunge leg to challenge your hip stability and strengthen your hip.
- You can rest your toe of the moving leg on the floor for support before moving again.

ADVANCED: When moving your leg back and forth, don't touch the floor. Try balancing in the lunge position while completing the set.

engaging your core on roller

Benefits: Strengthens your abdominal muscles (transverse, internal and external obliques, and rectus abdominis) while the roller supports your spine

STARTING POSITION: Lie lengthwise on the foam roller so your tailbone is at one end and your head is at the other. Bend your knees and place your feet hip-width apart on the floor. Place your arms by your sides so your palms touch the floor. Take a few breaths to get used to the unsteadiness.

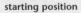

starting position

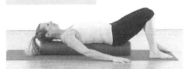

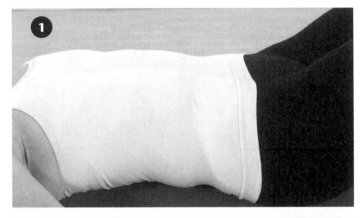

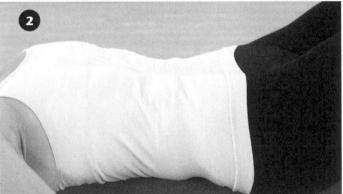

1–2 Inhale normally and then exhale fully to drop your belly button to the foam roller to strengthen your deep abdominal muscles.

Complete 5 breath cycles, inhaling for 3 counts, exhaling deeply for 5 counts. Eventually, you will increase the count to 5 inhalations and 8 exhalations.

TIPS

- Notice that when you engage your core muscles, you don't roll as much.

arm circles on roller

Benefits: Opens your chest and stretches your shoulders while challenging your core stability

STARTING POSITION: Lie lengthwise on the foam roller so your tailbone is at one end and your head is at the other. Bend your knees and place your feet hip-width apart on the floor. Place your arms by your sides so your palms touch the floor. Take a few breaths to get used to the unsteadiness.

starting position

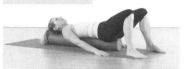

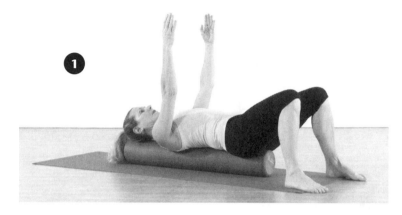

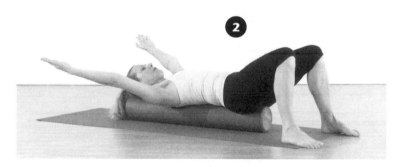

1 Raise your arms so your fingertips reach to the ceiling.

2 Lower your arms overhead, keeping your abdominals engaged so your back ribs remain on the roller.

3 Circle your arms down to your sides, palms up.

Circle 5 to 8 times and then reverse direction.

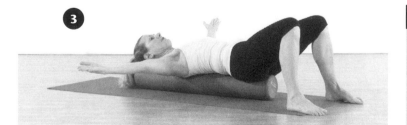

TIPS

- Don't let your back come off the roller—your back ribs must stay connected to the roller at all times.
- Engage your abdominals to help keep you stable on the roller as your arms circle.

moving arms on roller

Benefits: Strengthens your abdominal muscles (transverse, internal and external obliques, and rectus abdominis) as your arms challenge your core stability

STARTING POSITION: Lie lengthwise on the foam roller so your tailbone is at one end and your head is at the other. Bend your knees and place your feet hip-width apart on the floor. Place your arms by your sides so your palms touch the floor. Take a few breaths to get used to the unsteadiness.

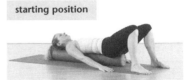

starting position

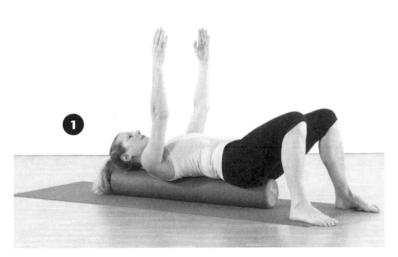

1 Raise your arms so your fingertips reach to the ceiling.

2 Inhale to lower your arms overhead, keeping your abdominals engaged so your back does not arch off the roller.

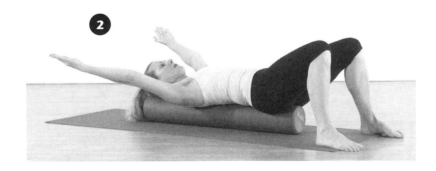

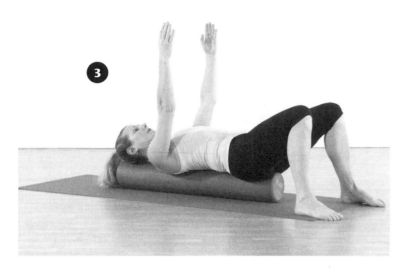

3 Exhale to move your arms to the ceiling again.

4 Hold this position and then lower down.

Complete 5 to 8 repetitions.

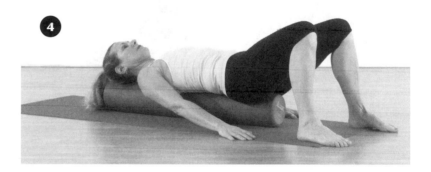

VARIATION: Instead of moving your arms in the same direction, you can also raise one arm as the other lowers.

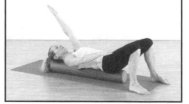

bent knees on roller

Benefits: Strengthens your abdominal muscles (transverse, internal and external obliques, and rectus abdominis) as your legs challenge your core stability

STARTING POSITION: Lie lengthwise on the foam roller so your tailbone is at one end and your head is at the other. Bend your knees and place your feet hip-width apart on the floor. Place your arms by your sides so your palms touch the floor. Take a few breaths to get used to the unsteadiness.

starting position

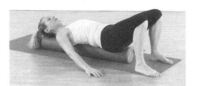

1

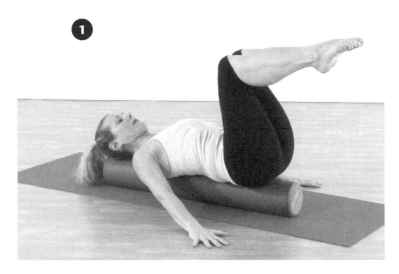

1 Bend your knees to a 90-degree angle, keeping your knees in line with your hip bones.

Complete 5 breath cycles, inhaling for 3 counts; exhaling deeply for 5 counts. Eventually, you will increase the count to 5 inhalations and 8 exhalations.

TIPS
• Focus on gently dropping your belly button to the roller to help keep you stable.

BEGINNER: If you feel too wobbly, just lift one leg while the other foot remains grounded on the floor.

Benefits: Strengthens your abdominal muscles (transverse, internal and external obliques, and rectus abdominis) as your legs challenge your core stability

STARTING POSITION: Lie lengthwise on the foam roller so your tailbone is at one end and your head is at the other. Bend your knees and place your feet hip-width apart on the floor. Place your arms by your sides so your palms touch the floor. Take a few breaths to get used to the unsteadiness.

starting position

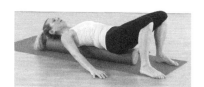

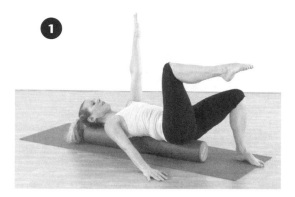

1 Lift your left arm so that your fingertips reach toward the ceiling and lift your right knee to a 90-degree angle, in line with your hip bones.

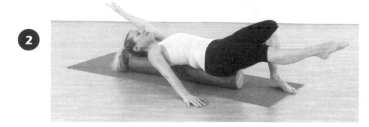

2 Inhale and, engaging your abs by pulling your belly button toward the roller, simultaneously lower your arm overhead and straighten your leg toward the floor.

3 Exhale deeply to raise both your arm and leg.

Repeat 5 to 8 times and then switch arm/leg.

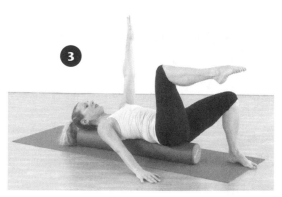

TIPS

• Focus on your exhale to help keep you steady.

toe dips on roller

Benefits: Strengthens your abdominal muscles (transverse, internal and external obliques, and rectus abdominis) as your legs challenge your core stability

STARTING POSITION: Lie lengthwise on the foam roller so your tailbone is at one end and your head is at the other. Bend your knees and place your feet hip-width apart on the floor. Place your arms by your sides so your palms touch the floor. Take a few breaths to get used to the unsteadiness.

starting position

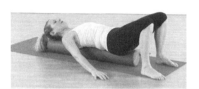

1 Bend your knees to a 90-degree angle.

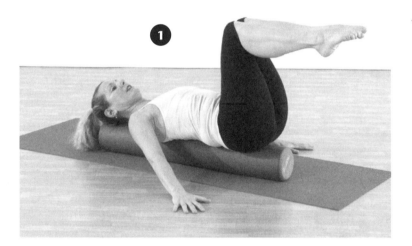

TIPS

- Melt your back ribs into the roller to strengthen your abs lengthen your back.
- Stabilize your pelvis so it does not move as your legs move. A deep exhale will help you maintain a neutral pelvis and stabilize your core.

- If you can't maintain proper alignment as you lower your toes, don't touch the floor with your toes—just move your legs enough to feel the belly challenge.

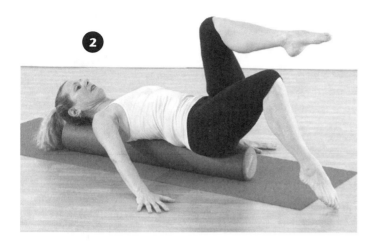

2 Inhale to lower your right toes to the floor, making sure that your belly button and back ribs remain on the roller.

3 Deeply exhale to bend your right leg to a 90-degree angle.

Repeat with the left leg. Continue alternating legs for 5 to 8 reps.

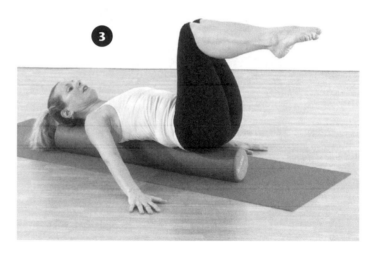

VARIATION: To advance this exercise, dip all ten toes to the floor rather than one foot at a time.

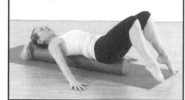

curl-down

Benefits: Strengthens your abdominal muscles (transverse, internal and external obliques, and rectus abdominis) while challenging your core stability

STARTING POSITION: Sit at one end of the roller, bending your knees and keeping your feet hip-width apart on the floor. Cross your hands and put your arms on your chest. Inhale to find your focus.

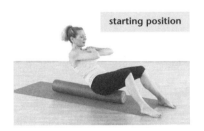

starting position

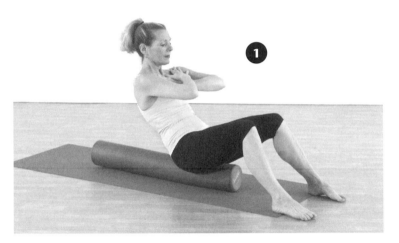

1

1 Exhale to slowly roll back one spinal bone at a time without using your hands. Focus on engaging your belly muscles. Only go down about 45 degrees or as far as you can go. After you complete the curl down, breathe normally to sit up any way you want.

Repeat 5 to 8 times.

TIPS

• Melt one bone of the spine at a time into the roller—think of lengthening from the base of your spine to the top of your head.

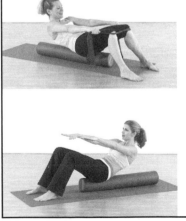

BEGINNER: If you have trouble articulating your spine, you can wrap an elastic band around both knees.

ADVANCED: Perform this exercise with your arms extended forward. From the curl-down position, try rolling up to a sitting position and then curling backdown. Inhale to roll up and then exhale to roll down.

straight legs on roller

Benefits: Strengthens your abdominal muscles (transverse, internal and external obliques, and rectus abdominis) as your legs challenge your core stability

The straight-leg position increases the stability challenge and puts more pressure on your lower back. Be careful!

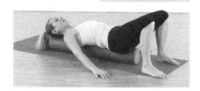

starting position

STARTING POSITION: Lie lengthwise on the foam roller so your tailbone is at one end and your head is at the other. Bend your knees and place your feet hip-width apart on the floor. Place your arms by your sides so your palms touch the floor. Take a few breaths to get used to the unsteadiness.

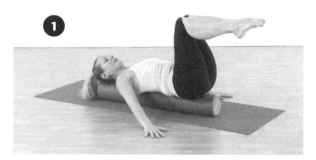

1 Bend your knees to a 90-degree angle.

2 Straighten your legs so your toes point to the ceiling. Focus on your exhale to engage your abs, dropping your belly button to the roller, to support your lower back.

Complete 5 breath cycles, inhaling for 3 counts, exhaling deeply for 5 counts. Eventually, you will increase the count to 5 inhalations and 8 exhalations

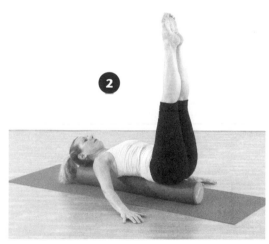

ADVANCED: For an extra challenge, lower your legs until they're 45 degrees from the floor.

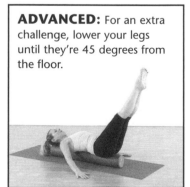

TIPS

• If you feel too wobbly, just lift one leg. Or if you can't straighten your legs, keep them slightly bent.

leg circle on roller

Benefits: Strengthens your abdominal muscles (transverse, internal and external obliques, and rectus abdominis) as your legs challenge your core stability

STARTING POSITION: Lie lengthwise on the foam roller so your tailbone is at one end, your head is at the other, and your legs are extended forward. Place your arms by your sides so your palms touch the floor. Take a few breaths to get used to the unsteadiness.

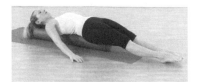

starting position

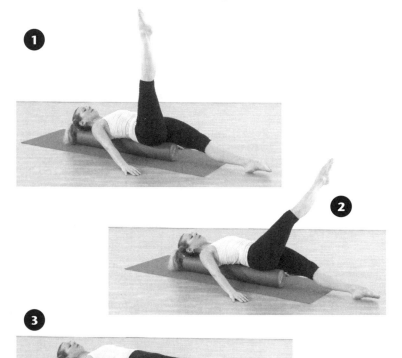

1 Lift your right leg so your toes point to ceiling; turn out your foot slightly.

2 Inhale and move your right toes toward your nose, then exhale to move your right leg across your body. Think about drawing a small circle on the ceiling with your big toe.

3 Continue to exhale and circle your right leg to your left heel and then up to the ceiling.

Repeat 5 leg circles and then reverse the direction. Switch legs.

TIPS

- Focus on dropping your belly button to the roller to help keep you steady.
- Make sure your leg is active and straight. If you can't straighten your leg, then bend the knee of the support leg.
- Continuously breathe as you swing your leg around to make a circle on the ceiling, focusing on your exhale to activate the deep stabilizing muscles of your core.

seated spinal twist with roller

Benefits: Strengthens your obliques plus cools off your back from the intense abdominal work of the roller exercises. The width of the roller will also help open your chest and stretch your shoulders.

Caution: If you have a lower back injury, please consult your doctor before doing this exercise or any rotation.

STARTING POSITION: Sit on your mat and straighten your legs, opening them hip-width apart. Place the roller between your back and underneath your arms, clasping loosely.

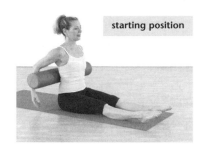
starting position

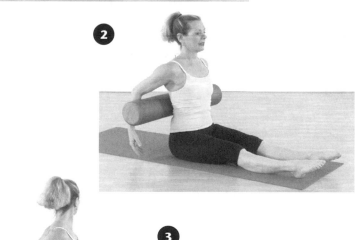

1 Inhale to grow tall through your spine, and then exhale to turn your body to the right. Rotate from the bottom ribs only. Remain stable in your lower back—nothing below your waist moves.

2 Inhale back to center.

3 Exhale to turn your body to the left.

Repeat 5 to 8 times.

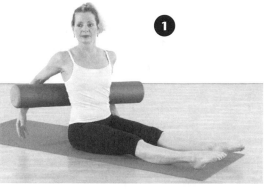

TIPS

- Initiate the rotation by growing tall in your spine, meaning sit as straight as possible.
- Focus on your exhale to tighten your ribs around your waist.
- If you can't straighten your legs, sit with your legs crossed or slightly bend your knees.

spinal extension on roller

Benefit: Stretches your ab muscles while strengthening your back muscles or spinal erectors. You may also feel a stretch across your shoulders.

STARTING POSITION: Lie on your stomach with your legs behind you. Place the roller under your forearms, halfway between your elbows and wrists, with the palms of your hands facing each other. Stretch your arms straight and rest your forehead on the floor.

starting position

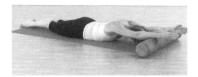

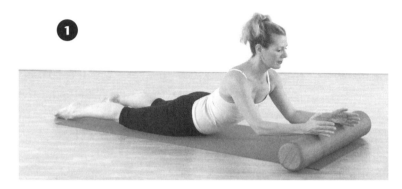

1 Inhale slowly to roll the roller toward your body and lift your chest, and then your abdomen, off the ground. Firm your glutes and hamstrings, press your pubic bone into the floor, and lift your belly button to your spine to protect your lower back. Gaze at the top of the roller so as not to strain your neck spinal bones.

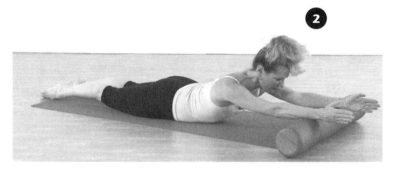

2 Exhale to roll the roller away from your body into the starting position.

Repeat 5 to 8 times.

TIPS

- Lift from the top of your head—imagine growing tall from your spine—and shift your chest forward to lengthen your back.
- If you feel discomfort in your lower back, don't lift your chest off the ground as high.

Focus on the principles: Draw your shoulder blades down your back, lengthen from the top of your head, and lift your breastbone as if a closed-fisted hand is pressing between your shoulder blades.

shoulder bridge on roller

Benefit: Strengthens your core muscles, hamstrings, and buttocks; stretches your hip flexors and quadriceps; challenges your core and hip stability

STARTING POSITION: Lie flat on your back, bend your knees, and place your feet on the roller. Keep your thighs parallel and even to engage your hamstrings and help your core muscles stay stable on the roller. Align your knees over your heels. Lengthen your arms by your sides, palms down, so you can press them into the floor. Make sure your body weight rests on your shoulders and upper back rather than your neck. Inhale to begin.

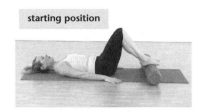

starting position

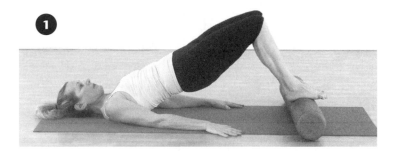

1 Exhale to lift your hips to the ceiling until your torso is off the ground.

2 Inhale to release down.

Complete 5 breath cycles, inhaling for 3 counts and exhaling deeply for 5 counts. Eventually, you will increase the count to 5 inhalations and 8 exhalations.

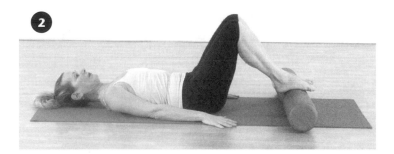

shoulder bridge on roller with leg lift and curl

Benefits: Strengthens your core muscles, hamstrings, and buttocks while challenging your core and hip stability

STARTING POSITION: Lie flat on your back with your knees bent and plant your heels into the center of the roller. Lengthen your arms by your sides, palms down, so you can press them into the floor to help lift and stabilize your torso as your legs work. Make sure your body weight rests on your shoulders and upper back rather than your neck. Inhale to begin.

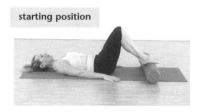

starting position

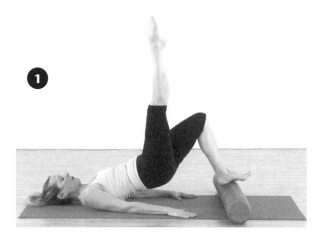

1 Straighten your right leg and lengthen your toes to the ceiling; focus on keeping your hips even and your pelvis stable to protect your lower back. Inhale to find your focus.

2 Exhale to slightly roll the roller toward your buttocks, using the heel of your left foot to control the roller while your pelvis continues to remain stable.

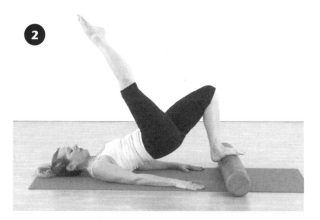

TIPS

- Don't drop the hip of the upper leg.
- Align your shoulders and pelvis so they form one line.
- Engage your core muscles by dropping your belly button to your spine.

plank on roller

Benefits: Strengthens your entire torso while challenging your total body stability: shoulders, hips, and core

STARTING POSITION: Place your hands shoulder-width apart on the roller; keep your elbows in line with your shoulders. Straighten your legs behind you, balancing on the balls of your feet so that your body is in a straight line from the top of your head to your heels. Draw your shoulder blades down your back, creating upper back and shoulder stability.

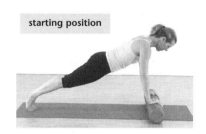
starting position

1

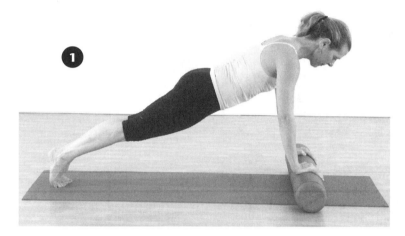

1 Hold for 30–60 seconds, lifting your belly button as if a string is lifting you up from the ceiling. Don't sag into your lower back.

2 After completing your breath work, sit your buttocks to your heels, as in a child's pose position.

2

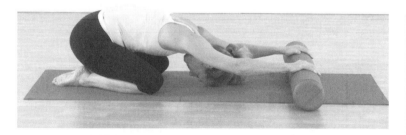

BEGINNER: Do this from a kneeling position, creating a diagonal line from the top of your head to your hips. Hold for 15 seconds, lifting your navel to your spine.

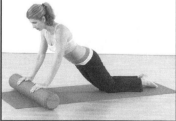

TIPS

• Engage your core muscles with each breath to help you stabilize and build core stability.

push-up on roller

Benefits: Strengthens your shoulders and chest muscles while challenging your total body stability: shoulders, hips, and core

STARTING POSITION: Place your hands, a littler wider than shoulder-width apart, on your roller. Straighten your legs behind you, balancing on the balls of your feet so that your body is in a straight line from the top of your head to your heels. Draw your shoulder blades down your back, creating upper back and shoulder stability. Lift your belly button to the sky.

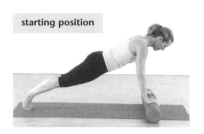

starting position

1

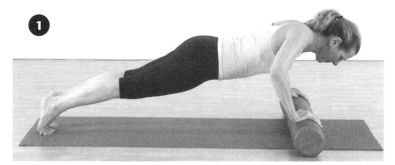

1 Inhale to maintain your plank as you bend your elbows, lowering your nose to the floor to a count of four. Move your elbows to the side to engage more chest muscles.

2

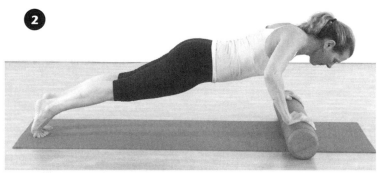

2 Exhale to push up your body to a plank position to a count of four.

TIPS

- If you don't have the strength to do a push-up, your upper back may sag, elevating your shoulders to your ears. Don't go down so low—only lower a little way and then push yourself up. Focus on good form.
- Head to heel like steel even as you lower yourself toward the floor—don't drop your head.

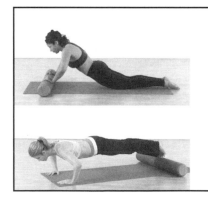

BEGINNER: Do this from a kneeling position, creating a diagonal line from the top of your head to your hips.

ADVANCED: Try the push-up by placing your toes on the roller and your hands on the floor; point your fingertips in slightly. Make sure to maintain the plank position.

reverse crunch on roller

Benefits: Strengthens your core muscles while challenging your total body stability: shoulders, hips, and core

This is an advanced exercise.

STARTING POSITION: Put the tops of your feet on the roller and then place your hands on the floor in front of the roller. Walk your hands out until you're in a straight line. Align your wrists directly under your shoulders; your arms can be slightly bent. Look at the floor to lengthen your neck. Inhale to find your core stability.

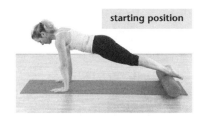
starting position

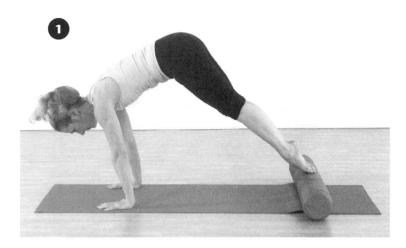

1 Exhale deeply to lift your hips to the sky, forcing your abs into action as you move into a slight pike position. Your hips don't have to lift too high—just enough to feel your abs contract.

2 Inhale back into plank position.

Repeat 5 to 8 times.

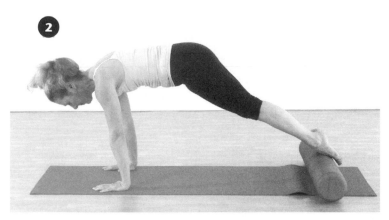

seated ball: finding neutral spine

Benefits: Strengthens your abdominal muscles (transverse, internal and external obliques, and rectus abdominis); challenges core stability; warms up the spine

STARTING POSITION: Sit your butt bones, located under the cheeky portion of your bottom, on top of your ball. Keep your knees hip-width apart, feet parallel and firmly grounded on the floor. Place your hands on your thighs and align your shoulders directly over your hips. Inhale to sit tall, lengthening your spine.

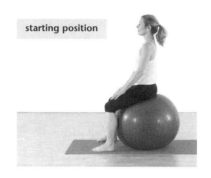

starting position

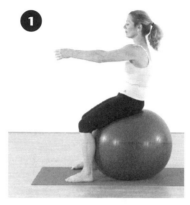

1

1 Exhale to raise your arms parallel to the floor and slowly tip your pubic bone to the ceiling, moving your navel closer to your spine and allowing the ball to roll forward.

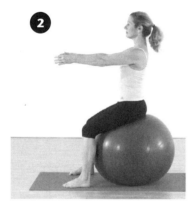

2

2 Inhale to return to a neutral spine, sitting tall in your spine.

3 Exhale to slowly move your pubic bone to the floor while your lower back arches, allowing the ball to roll behind you.

Return to a neutral spine.

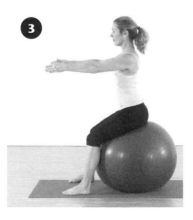

3

TIPS

• Engage your abs by lifting your belly button up and in under your rib cage toward your spine.

• If you feel very shaky, make your movements very small.

ball bridge

Benefits: Strengthens your core muscles, hamstrings, and buttocks; stretches your hip flexors and quadriceps; challenges your core and hip stability

STARTING POSITION: Sit on the center of your ball.

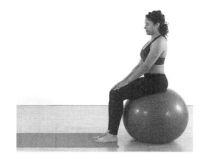

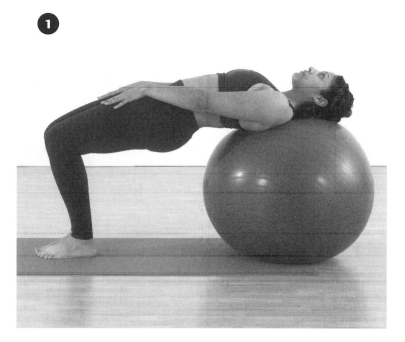

1

1 Walk your feet forward until your upper back and neck are on the ball. Place your hands on your thighs. In one motion, lift your hips to the ceiling so your thighs are parallel to the floor.

Complete 5 to 8 breath cycles, inhaling for 3 counts, exhaling deeply for 5 counts. Return to sitting position.

ball bridge with arm circles

Benefits: Opens your chest, stretches your shoulders, challenges your core and hip stability

STARTING POSITION: Sit on the center of your ball and then walk your feet forward until your upper back and neck are on the ball. Gently curl your chin to your chest to lengthen and protect your neck and spine. Your thighs are parallel to the floor and your hip bones are even. Align your hips with your knees and your knees directly over your ankles. Place your hands on your thighs. Keep your body weight in your heels to activate your buttocks.

starting position

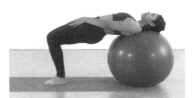

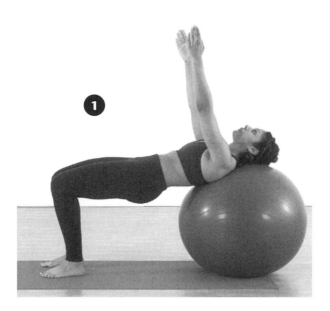

1 Raise your arms, lifting your fingertips toward the ceiling.

TIPS

- Place your head and upper back on the ball—don't let your head hang off the ball.
- Engage your core muscles to keep your bottom from dropping to the floor.

- Don't place your feet too close to the ball—this can strain your knees.
- If you feel wobbly, place your fingertips on the floor to help stabilize you.

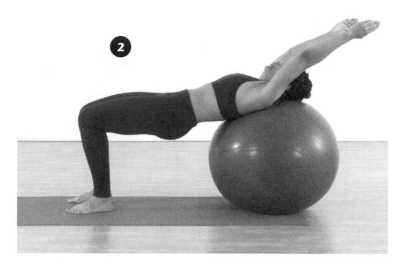

2 Inhale to lower your arms over your head, keeping your abdominals contracted to the ball so that your back does not arch.

3 Exhale to circle your arms to your sides, palms up, continuing the circle until your fingertips are reaching to the ceiling.

Return to sitting position.

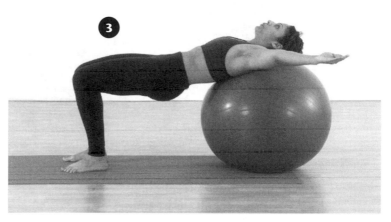

ADVANCED: Add 2 or 3lb. dumbbell weights to increase the intensity of the stretch and core and hip stability challenge.

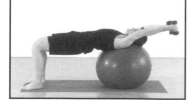

abdominal ball curl

Benefits: Strengthens your abdominal muscles (transverse, internal and external obliques, and rectus abdominis) while challenging your core stability

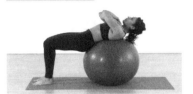

STARTING POSITION: Sit on the center of your ball and then walk your feet forward until your back and shoulders are on the ball. Place your feet parallel and align your knees hip-width apart; firmly ground your feet on the floor. Place your hands on your chest, crossing them at your wrists. Inhale to begin.

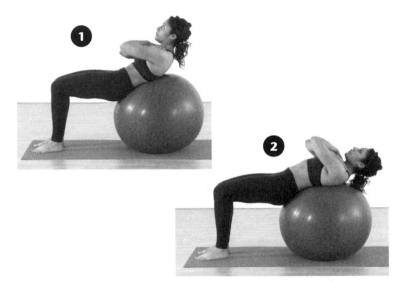

1 Exhale to curl your chin to your chest and lift your shoulders off the ball about three inches. Pull your ribs to your hips to engage your abs.

2 Inhale to starting position.

INTERMEDIATE: To increase the stability challenge, move your feet closer together, decreasing your base of support.

ADVANCED: Do the exercise by holding one 8 or 10lb. dumbbell on your chest.

EXTREME: For an extreme challenge, do the advanced exercise with your arms extended above your head.

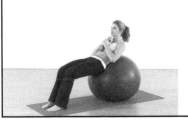

TIPS

- Gently guide your chin to your chest to lengthen the back of your neck and avoid straining your neck muscles.
- Exhale deeply to engage your transverse, creating a bracing sensation around your waist.
- Don't bounce into position—use your abs to lift and lower your torso off the ball.
- Use your legs to steady the ball.

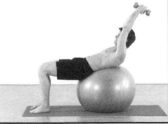

abdominal oblique ball curl

Benefits: Strengthens your internal and external oblique abdominals while challenging your core stability

starting position

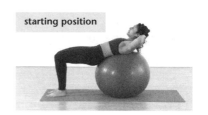

STARTING POSITION: Sit on the center of your ball, feet parallel and firmly grounded on the floor. Walk your feet away from the ball until your lower back presses against the ball. Interlace your fingers and place your hands loosely behind your head for neck support. Don't pull on your head, which can create neck tension. Keep your elbows out to the side throughout the exercise. Inhale to begin.

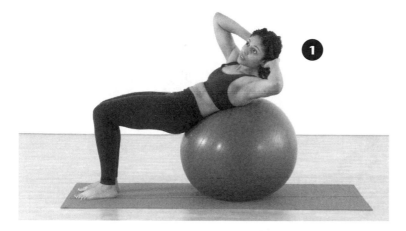

1

1 Exhale deeply to lift your torso off the ball and then turn your chest to the left so that your right elbow crosses your left thigh and your ribs move to your hips. Keep your lower back anchored to the ball.

2 Inhale to lower your body to the ball.

Repeat to the other side.

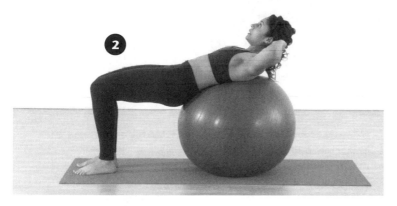

2

TIPS

• As you twist, initiate rotation from your bottom ribs.
• Use your elbow to increase the intensity of the twist.

ADVANCED: To increase the stability challenge, bring your feet closer together.

spinal extension on ball

Benefit: Stretches your ab muscles while strengthening your back muscles or spinal erectors

Caution: If you have a lower back injury, please check with your doctor before attempting any level of spinal extension.

STARTING POSITION: Balancing on the balls of your feet, drape yourself over the ball. Wrap your arms around the ball as you curl your chest, abdomen, and hips over it. Gaze at the floor to align your neck with your spine.

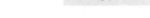

starting position

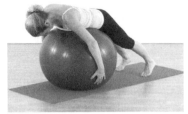

1

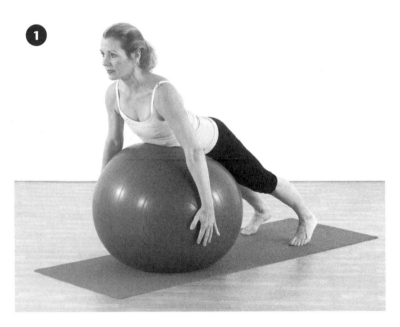

1 Inhale to lift your chest off the ball, straightening your spine. Focus on your shoulders, making sure they don't rise toward your ears.

Exhale to lower.

INTERMEDIATE: Try placing your hands on the backs of your thighs.

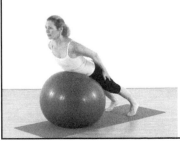

ADVANCED: For an intense challenge, raise your arms by your ears, but make sure to keep your shoulders down.

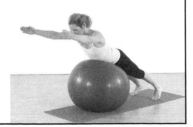

TIPS
- Lengthen from the top of your head so you don't put needless pressure on your lower back.
- Keep your hands close to your body.

spinal cross-extension on ball

Benefits: Strengthens your back muscles as you learn to stabilize your spine against the weight of your limbs

Caution: If you have a lower back injury, please consult your doctor before attempting a spinal extension.

STARTING POSITION: Rest your belly and your upper thighs on the ball. You can place your hands on the floor for support. Gaze at the floor.

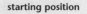
starting position

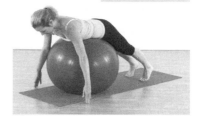

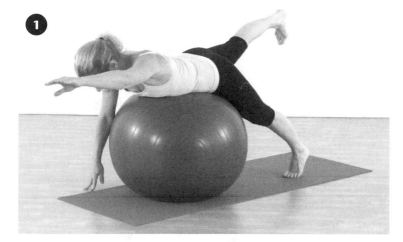

1

1 Simultaneously lift your left arm and right leg, moving from the heel to engage your buttock muscles. Maintain a stable pelvis and keep your hip bones even—don't lift your leg higher than your torso. Hold this contraction for 5 to 8 breaths.

2 Lower your limbs to starting position.

After 3 sets, repeat on the opposite side of your body.

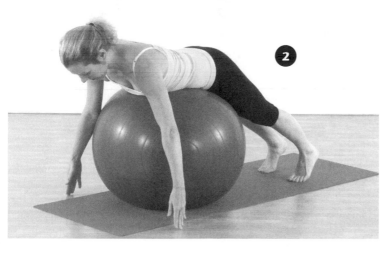

2

TIPS

- Lift your belly button to your navel to support your back.
- Don't lift or drop your head—keep your head in line with your spine to lengthen it.

one-legged lunge with ball

Benefits: Strengthens all of the muscles in your legs and hips, including your buttocks; challenges your total body stability

STARTING POSITION: Stand in front of your ball with your feet hip-width apart. Place the top of your right foot on the ball so that your thigh is perpendicular to the floor. Straighten your arms by your sides, fingertips lengthening to the floor. Maintain spinal stability by lifting your breastbone to help lengthen and lift your spine.

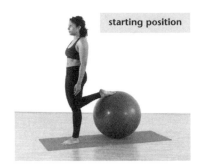

starting position

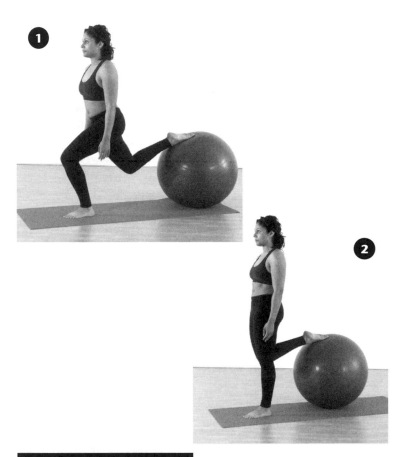

1 Bend the standing leg and roll the ball behind you, guiding it with your foot so that the standing leg is in a deep lunge with the thigh almost parallel to the floor. Point your hip bones toward the floor, keeping them as even as possible.

2 Stay in your lunge to inhale. Then exhale to roll the ball in. Align the knee of your standing leg directly over the heel of your foot.

Repeat 5 to 8 times and then switch legs.

TIPS

• Sit into your thigh as you lunge to activate more hip muscles and challenge your hip stability.

BEGINNER: If you feel very unstable, place your fingertips on a wall for support. To get in the best position, measure an arm's length from the wall and stand there.

one-legged deadlift with ball

Benefits: Strengthens the muscles of your legs, especially your hamstrings, while challenging your total body stability

STARTING POSITION: Stand with your feet hip-width apart and hold your ball. Maintain spinal stability by lifting your breastbone to help lengthen and lift your spine. Straighten your arms in front of you, lengthening your fingertips. Gaze at your ball.

starting position

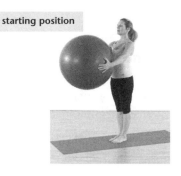

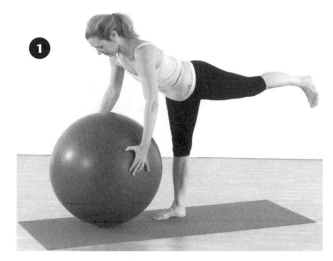

1 Inhale to slowly lift your right leg behind you, lifting from your heel to engage your buttocks and hamstrings, as you lower your torso to the ground. Maintain your hip alignment, making sure your hip points face down and are even. Stop when your head, torso, and leg are in a straight line and parallel to the floor.

2 Exhale to slowly lower your leg to the floor and return to standing.

Repeat 5 to 8 times and then switch legs.

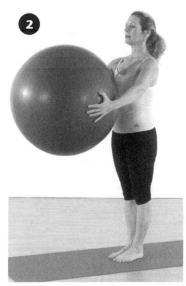

TIPS

- Engage your core muscles to help stabilize your inner thighs and keep your hips even.
- Engage your inner thighs to keep your hips even.

one-legged standing row and deadlift with ball

Benefits: Strengthens your triceps and the muscles of your back, such as your lats, while challenging your total body stability

STARTING POSITION: Stand to the left of your ball and place your fingertips on it. Hold an 8 to 10lb. dumbbell in your left hand and straighten your arm to the floor, keeping your palm in and making sure your hand is in line with your shoulder. Lift your left leg so that it's parallel to the floor. Lengthen from the top of your head to your foot to help keep you balanced.

starting position

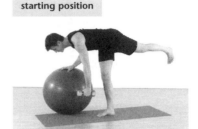

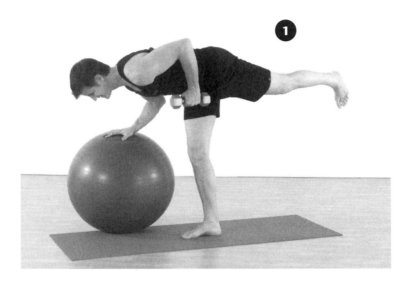

1 Inhale to bend your elbow and lift the back of your arm to the ceiling. The dumbbell slides past your rib cage as your elbow lifts high to the ceiling.

2 Exhale to lower the dumbbell to the floor.

Repeat 5 to 8 times. Switch leg and arm.

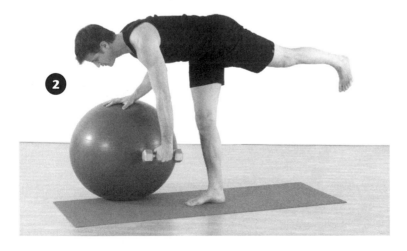

TIPS

- It's okay if the standing leg's knee is slightly bent.
- Lift the pit of your belly to the ceiling to help support your back, strengthen your core, and keep you steady.
- Engage your inner thighs to keep your hips even.

triceps kickback

Benefits: Strengthens your triceps and the muscles of your back, such as your lats, while challenging your total body stability

STARTING POSITION: Stand to the left of your ball and place your fingertips on it. Hold an 8 to 10lb. dumbbell weight in your left hand and straighten your arm to the floor, keeping your palm in and making sure your hand is in line with your shoulder. Lift your left leg so that it's parallel to the floor and straighten your right leg. Lengthen from the top of your head to your foot to help keep you balanced.

starting position

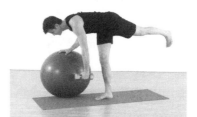

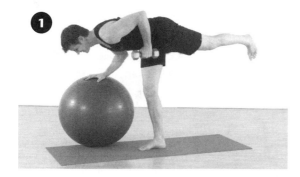

1 Inhale to bend your elbow and lift the back of your arm to the ceiling. The dumbbell weight slides past your rib cage as your elbow lifts high to the ceiling.

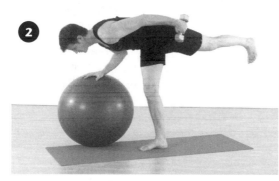

2 Slowly straighten your arm behind you.

3 Exhale to the starting position.

Repeat 5 to 8 times and then switch leg and arm.

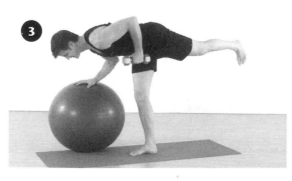

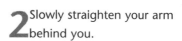
TIPS

- It's okay if the standing leg's knee is slightly bent.
- Lift the pit of your belly to the ceiling to help support your back, strengthen your core, and keep you steady.
- Engage your inner thighs to keep your hips even.

plank on ball

Benefits: Strengthens your upper back muscles while challenging your total body stability (hips, core, and shoulders)

STARTING POSITION: Lie on your ball, rounding your chest, abdomen, and hips over it. Place your hands on the floor in front of the ball.

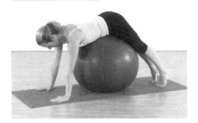

starting position

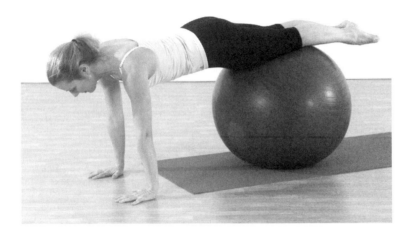

1 Walk your hands out until the ball rolls near your hips and your legs are straight. Place your hands directly under your shoulders to build strength and reinforce proper upper back alignment. Draw your shoulder blades down your back, creating upper back and shoulder stability. Hold for 30 seconds, focusing on exhaling to lift your navel to the ceiling to strengthen your core stability.

After completing your breath work, hug your ball.

TIPS

- If you feel any lower back strain, focus on your hip and core alignment. Lift your navel to your spine and engage your abs to protect your back. If that doesn't relieve the discomfort, stop this exercise.
- Don't let your upper back arch. Slide your shoulder blades down your back to create shoulder and upper back stability.
- Don't lift your shoulders to your ears.

BEGINNER: To lessen the intensity, roll the ball until it's near your abdomen. Hold for 15 seconds.

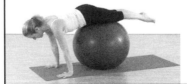

ADVANCED: To increase the challenge, place your feet on the ball and then walk your hands out until you are in a straight line. Make sure to place your hands directly under your shoulders and draw your shoulder blades down your back. Hold for 60 seconds, lifting your navel to your spine.

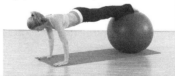

ball bridge on floor

Benefits: Strengthens your buttocks and hamstrings while challenging your core and hip stability

STARTING POSITION: Lie on your back with the ball under your knees so that it touches the backs of your thighs. Straighten your arms by your sides, lengthening your fingertips to your toes.

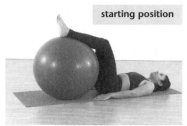
starting position

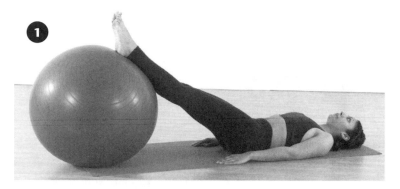

1 Walk the ball away from your bottom so that it rests against your calves.

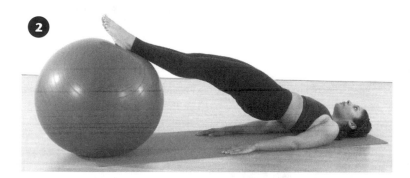

2 In one movement, lift your hips to the ceiling. Hold this Bridge for 5 to 8 breaths.

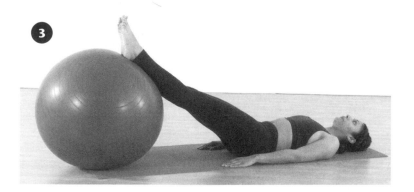

3 Lower your spine slowly to the floor, roll the ball back under the backs of your thighs, and relax.

ball bridge with leg lift

Benefits: Strengthens your buttocks and hamstrings while challenging your core and hip stability

STARTING POSITION: Lie on your back with the ball under your knees so it touches the backs of your thighs. Straighten your arms by your sides, lengthening your fingertips to your toes. Press the palms of your hands into the floor to help lift and stabilize your torso.

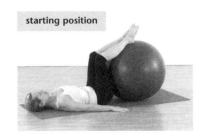

starting position

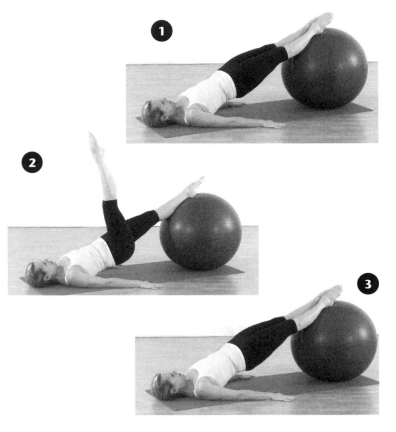

1 Roll the ball away from your bottom so that it rests against your calves and then lift your hips off the floor. Plant your heels into the center of your ball. Align your shoulders and pelvis so that they are even and stable to create total body stability.

2 Inhale to lift from your buttocks muscles to kick your right leg up toward the ceiling; focus on keeping your hips even and your pelvis stable to prevent your hip from drooping.

3 Exhale to lower the leg back to the ball.

Repeat 5 to 8 times and then switch legs.

TIPS

- Engage your core muscles, exhaling deeply to create brace-like support for your torso.
- When you lower your spine to the floor, do so with control, focusing on each bone of your spine.

Benefits: Strengthens your buttocks and hamstrings while challenging your core and hip stability

STARTING POSITION: Lie on your back with the ball under your calves and then lift your hips off the floor. Straighten your arms by your sides, lengthening your fingertips to your toes. Press the palms of your hands into the floor to help lift and stabilize your torso.

starting position

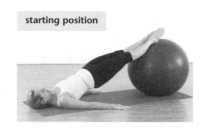

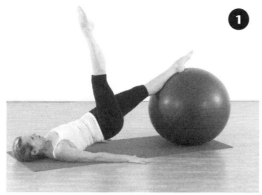

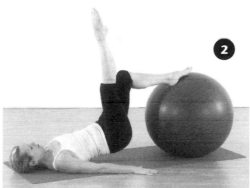

1 Lift your right leg toward the ceiling, lengthening your toes.

2 In one motion, bend your left knee and inhale to roll the ball toward your buttocks.

3 Exhale to roll the ball away from your butt. Keep your hips lifted. You are simultaneously lifting your leg while the other leg does a leg curl.

Repeat 5 to 8 times and then switch legs.

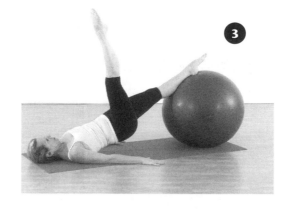

TIPS

- Engage your core muscles— exhaling deeply to create a brace-like support for your torso.
- When you lower your spine to the floor, do so with control, focusing on each bone of your spine.

pike on ball

Benefits: Strengthens your upper back muscles and abs while challenging your total body stability (hips, core, and shoulders)

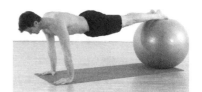

STARTING POSITION: Kneel in front of your ball and round your chest, abdomen, and hips over it. Place your hands on the floor in front of the ball. Walk your hands out until your feet are on the ball. You're in a plank position, forming a straight line with your body. Make sure your hands are directly under your shoulders and activate your abs by lifting your belly button to the ceiling to strengthen your core stability.

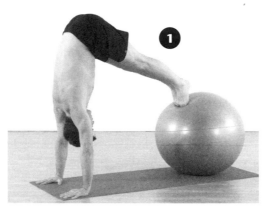

1 Inhale and then exhale to lift your hips to the sky so that your body forms an upside-down "V." Remember to keep your shoulders away from your ears.

2 Inhale to return to starting position.

Repeat 5 to 8 times.

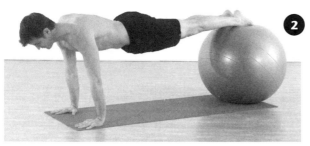

TIPS

- If you feel any lower back strain, focus on your hip and core alignment. Lift your navel to your spine and engage your abs to protect your back. If that doesn't relieve the discomfort, stop this exercise.
- Align your hands so they are directly underneath your shoulders to build strength and reinforce proper upper back alignment.
- Don't let your upper back arch. Slide your shoulder blades down your back to create shoulder and upper back stability.

push-up on ball

Benefits: Strengthens your shoulders and chest muscles while challenging your total body stability (shoulders, hips, and core)

STARTING POSITION: Kneel in front of your ball and round your chest, abdomen, and hips over it. Place your hands on the floor in front of the ball. Walk your hands out until the ball rolls near your hips and your legs are straight. Place your hands a littler wider than shoulder-width apart and lift your belly button to the ceiling.

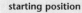

starting position

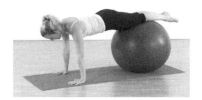

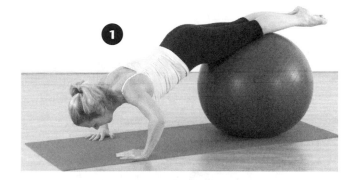

1 To a count of four, maintain your plank as you bend your elbows, inhaling to lower your nose to the floor. Allow your elbows to move to the side to engage more chest muscles.

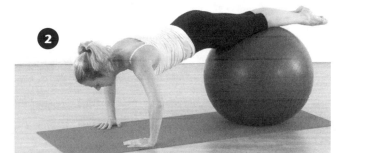

2 Counting to four, exhale to push up until your body is back in the plank position.

TIPS

- If you don't have the strength to do a push-up, your upper back may sag, elevating your shoulders to your ears. Don't go down so low—only lower a little way and then push yourself up. Focus on good form.
- Head to heel like steel even as you lower toward the floor.

BEGINNER: To lessen the intensity, walk your hands out until the ball rolls near your abdomen.

ADVANCED: To increase the challenge, place your feet on the ball and then walk your hands out until you are in a straight line.

ball pike and push-up combination

Benefits: Strengthens your chest and abs while challenging your total body stability (shoulders, hips, and core)

This is an advanced exercise.

STARTING POSITION: Kneel in front of your ball and round your chest, abdomen, and hips over it. Place your hands on the floor in front of the ball. Walk your hands out until you're in a plank position, with your feet on the ball and your body forming a straight line. Place your hands directly under your shoulders.

starting position

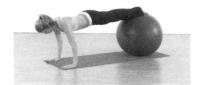

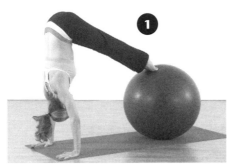

1 Inhale to find your core stability and then exhale to lift your hips to the sky so that your body forms an upside-down "V."

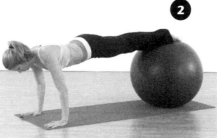

2 Inhale to lower back down into the plank position.

3 Exhale as you bend your elbows, lowering your nose to the floor to do a push-up.

Repeat 5 to 8 times.

TIPS

- Move with control and use your breath to force your abs into action.
- Exhale to squeeze out every ounce of strength from your abs and support your lower back in the plank position.
- Don't drop your head—instead, lengthen from the top to make a straight line with your body.

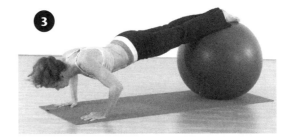

ball plank with foam roller

Benefits: Strengthens your shoulders and core muscles while challenging your total body stability (shoulders, core, and hips)

Here you work against two unstable points, which makes this exercise very advanced.

STARTING POSITION: Kneel behind your ball and round your chest, abdomen, and hips over it. Place your hands on the roller and roll yourself forward until your feet are on the ball and your body forms a straight line. Make sure your hands are directly under your shoulders and draw your shoulder blades down your back, creating upper back and shoulder stability.

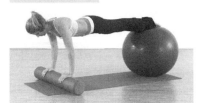

starting position

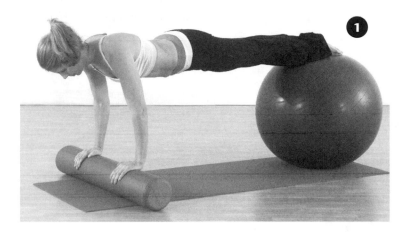

1 Find your focus and hold for 30–60 seconds, lifting your navel to your spine to strengthen your core stability.

TIPS

- If you feel any lower back strain, focus on your hip and core alignment. Lift your navel to your spine and engage your abs to protect your back. If that doesn't relieve the discomfort, then stop this exercise.
- Align your hands so they are directly underneath your shoulders to build strength and reinforce proper upper back alignment.
- Don't let your upper back arch.
- Don't lift your shoulders to your ears.

EXTREME: For an even greater challenge, place your elbows on the roller.

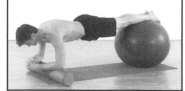

drape over ball

Benefits: Soothes your muscles and eases tension in your back.

A great way to end a ball workout! It's also wonderful to do after a long day of sitting or standing.

STARTING POSITION: Kneel in front of your ball and round your chest, abdomen, and hips over it.

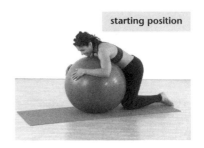

starting position

1 Roll the ball under your belly, relaxing and focusing on deep breathing.

1

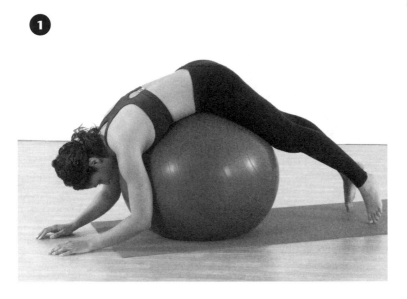

Benefits: Strengthens your core muscles while developing shoulder and pelvis stability

STARTING POSITION: With the balance board held lengthwise, place the balance board in front of your right knee and place your right hand on the board. Breathe normally.

starting position

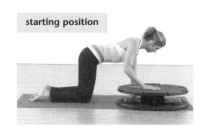

1

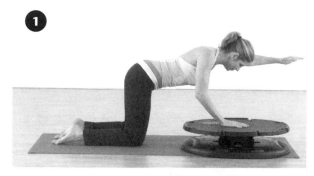

2

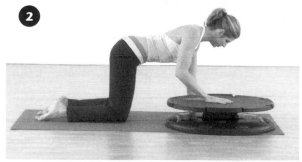

1 Focus on exhaling deeply to lift your abs to your spine yet keeping a flat back and stable pelvis; lift your left hand off the floor.

2 Lower it back to the board.

Repeat.

TIPS

- Lengthen from the top of your head to your tailbone.
- Activate your upper back muscles by sliding your shoulder blades down your back.

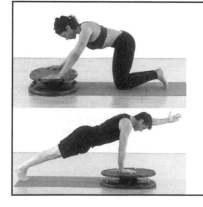

BEGINNER: Kneel in front of your balance board and place both hands on it. Make sure your arms are directly under your shoulders and your knees are directly under your hip bones. Complete 5 breath cycles.

ADVANCED: Try this with your legs straight for an extra challenge.

spinal cross-extension on balance board

Benefits: Strengthens your back muscles while focusing on activating your deep abdominals, such as the transverse

STARTING POSITION: While kneeling, place the balance board in front of your right knee and place your right hand on the board. Breathe normally but focus on your exhale to lift your abdominals to your spine, engaging your deep abdominals to support your lower back and keep your steady.

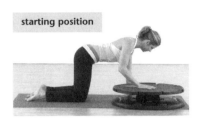

starting position

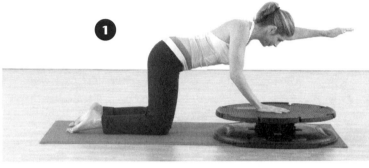

1 Lift your left hand off the floor.

2 Slowly lifting the heel of your right foot to the ceiling, raise your leg until it's straight and even with your buttocks.

After 5 to 8 breaths, switch legs and hands.

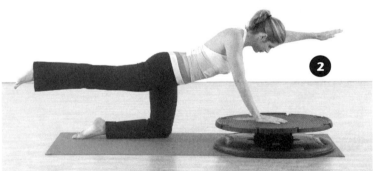

TIPS

- Keep your back flat even though you're lifting your abs to your spine.
- Try to feel your waist shrink with every exhale.

INTERMEDIATE: Inhale to straighten both your arm and leg simultaneously and then exhale to return to starting position.

ADVANCED: For an intense core challenge, straighten your legs.

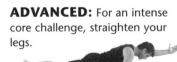

bridge on BOSU

Benefits: Strengthens your core muscles and several muscle groups of your backside while challenging your hip stability

starting position

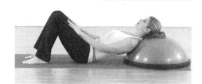

STARTING POSITION: Sit on the center of your BOSU and then walk your feet forward until your upper back and neck are on it—make sure your head does not hang off. Gently curl your chin to your chest to lengthen and protect your neck and spine. Place your hands on your thighs.

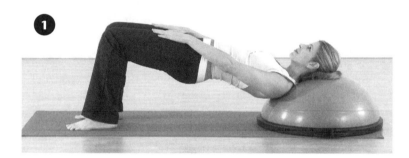

1 In one motion, lift your hips to the ceiling so your thighs are parallel to the floor. Your knees should also be parallel and at a 90-degree angle, aligned directly over your ankles. Make sure your hip bones are even as you complete 5 to 8 breath cycles, inhaling for 3 counts, exhaling deeply for 5 counts.

Return to sitting position.

INTERMEDIATE: While your hips are lifted to the ceiling, raise your fingers to the ceiling.

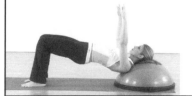

ADVANCED: While your hips are lifted to the ceiling, slowly kick your left leg up and move your right arm across your body. Your right leg maintains a 90-degree angle and is parallel to the floor.

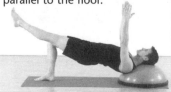

TIPS

- Keep your body weight in your heels to activate your buttocks.
- Engage your core muscles to keep your butt from dropping to the floor.

spinal extension on balance cushion

Benefits: Strengthens your back muscles, or the erector spinae that run lengthwise along your spine

Caution: If you have a lower back injury, please check with your doctor before attempting any level of spinal extension.

STARTING POSITION: Lie face down and place your balance cushion under your abdomen, between your belly button and pelvis. Gently lift your belly button to your spine to support your back. Cross your hands and place your palms under your forehead and on the floor. Gaze at the floor to align your neck with your spine.

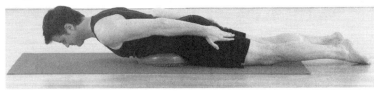

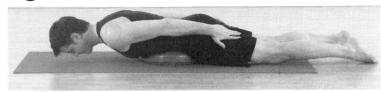

1 Inhale to reach your arms along your sides and lift your chest off the ground, lengthening your spine. Focus on relaxing your shoulders so they don't elevate toward your ears as you lift. Firm your buttocks and hamstrings to protect your lower back. Hold for 3 to 5 breaths.

2 Lower down to starting position.

Repeat 5 times.

TIPS

• Lengthen from the top of your head so that you don't put needless pressure on your lower back.

ADVANCED: To increase the challenge, straighten your arms and legs and then inhale to lift your chest off the ground. Hold for 5 to 8 breaths. Repeat 5 to 8 times.

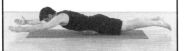

spinal cross-extension on cushion (swimming)

Benefits: Strengthens your back muscles as you learn to stabilize your spine against the movement of your limbs

Caution: If you have a lower back injury, please consult your doctor before attempting any spinal extension.

STARTING POSITION: Lie face down and place your balance cushion under your abdomen, between your belly button and pelvis. Your arms and legs are straight and active; firm your buttocks and hamstrings to protect your lower back. Gaze at the floor, keeping your head in line with your spine to lengthen it.

starting position

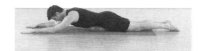

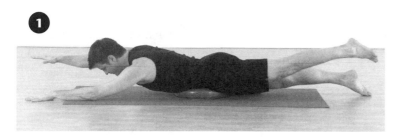

1 Simultaneously lift your right leg and left arm, lifting from your heel to engage your hamstrings and buttock muscles. Gently lift your belly button to your spine to support your back. Hold this contraction for 5 to 8 breaths.

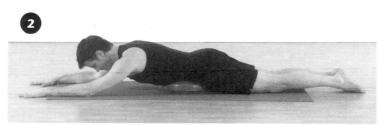

2 Lower your limbs to the floor.

Do 5 sets, then repeat on the opposite side.

TIPS

- Your limbs are challenging your stability; therefore, maintain a stable pelvis.
- Align your legs with your torso; lifting your legs any higher can throw you off balance.
- Don't lift or drop your head.

ADVANCED: Lift your right leg and left arm, but instead of holding them in place, lower and raise your left leg and right arm. Continue alternating the lifting and lowering movements as if you're swimming. Breathe normally. Do 5 to 8 reps.

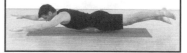

plank on balance board

Benefits: Strengthens your core and shoulder muscles while challenging your total body stability

STARTING POSITION: Kneel in front of your balance board and place your hands a little wider than shoulder-width apart on the edges of it.

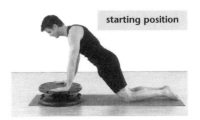
starting position

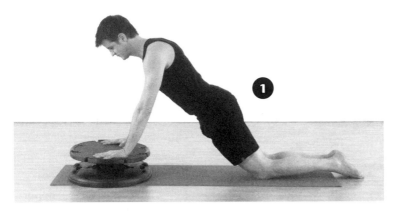
①

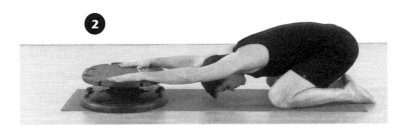
②

1 Walk your hips away from the balance board so you can get into a plank position on your knees. Lower your hips so that they are in line with your torso. Draw your shoulder blades down your back, creating upper back and shoulder stability. No sagging in the middle—engage your abs. Hold for 15 seconds, lifting your navel to your spine.

2 After completing your breath work, sit your buttocks to your heels, as in a child's pose position.

ADVANCED: To increase the challenge, do this in a plank position with your legs straight, forming a straight line with your body. Hold for 30–60 seconds.

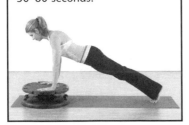

TIPS

- Use your exhale to activate your abs by lifting your belly button to the ceiling (but maintaining a flat table-top back) for core stability.
- If you feel any lower back strain, focus on your hip and core alignment. Lift your navel to your spine to support your lower back. If this doesn't relieve the discomfort, then stop this exercise.
- Don't let your back arch.
- Don't lift your shoulders to your ears.

cross-extension plank on balance board

Benefits: Strengthens your core, shoulder, and leg muscles while challenging your total body stability

Caution: This is an advanced exercise. If you have a shoulder injury, don't do this plank.

STARTING POSITION: Place the balance board lengthwise in front of your left knee. Place your left hand on the board directly under your shoulder; draw your shoulder blades down your back, creating upper back and shoulder stability. Straighten your legs so that you're in a plank position. Gaze at the floor.

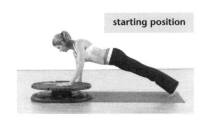

starting position

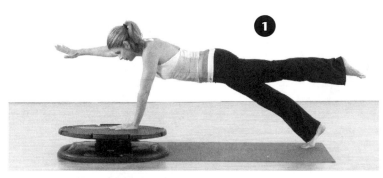

1 Simultaneously raise your right arm and left leg slowly, lifting from your heel to engage your buttock muscles. Your arm and leg on the opposite side should be in a straight line. Focus on maintaining a neutral spine, with your hip bones even and pointed toward the floor. Hold this position for 5 to 8 breaths.

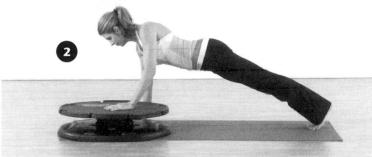

2 Lower your limbs to the floor.

Do 3 sets, and then repeat on the opposite side.

TIPS

- Use your breath to engage your abs to support your back.
- To help create stability, lengthen your limbs from your core to activate as many muscles as possible.
- Lengthen from the top of your head, keeping your head in line with your spine.

side plank on BOSU

Benefits: Strengthens the muscles of the waist such as abdominal obliques and quadratus lumborum; challenges your total body stability

STARTING POSITION: Sit on your right side with your knees slightly pulled into your body, stacked on top of each other. Place your elbow on the BOSU directly under your shoulder.

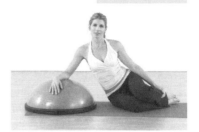

starting position

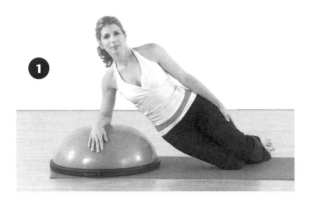

1

1 In one motion, lift your torso, hips, and thighs off the floor so you are balancing on your elbow and the side of your knee. Rest your free arm on the side of your body. Don't sag into your shoulder or waist; lift from your hips as if a string from the ceiling were pulling you up. Hold for 15 seconds, breathing normally.

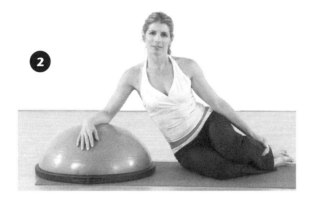

2

2 Lower down to starting position and switch sides.

TIPS

• Engage your core muscles on each breath to help you stabilize.

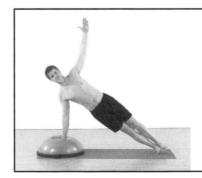

ADVANCED: To increase the challenge, place your hand in the center of the BOSU and straighten your legs so you are now balancing on your hand and the side of your foot. Lift your top arm to the ceiling, lengthening from your fingertips. Hold for 30 seconds.

one-arm elbow plank on BOSU

Benefits: Strengthens your core while challenging your total body stability

STARTING POSITION: Kneel in front of your BOSU and place your elbows shoulder-width apart on the dome.

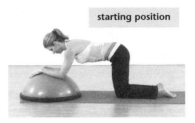
starting position

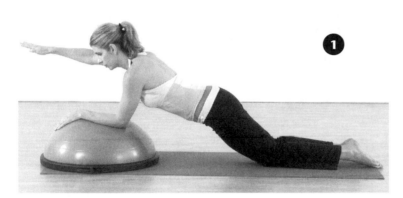

1 Walk your hips away from the BOSU so you can get into a plank position on your knees and then lower your hips so they are in line with your torso. Draw your shoulder blades down your back, creating upper back and shoulder stability. Breathe normally. Slowly lift your right elbow off the BOSU and straighten your arm to the front.

2 Return your elbow to the BOSU and switch arms.

ADVANCED: You can also do this so that your legs are straight and you're balancing on the balls of your feet.

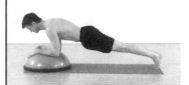 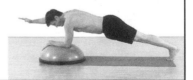

bridge on floor with balance board

Benefits: Strengthens your core, hamstrings, and buttocks while challenging your hip and core stability

STARTING POSITION: Lie on your back with the balance board under your feet; your knees are parallel and bent at a 90-degree position. Keep your hands out to the sides, pressing the palms of your hands into the floor to help lift and stabilize your torso as your legs work.

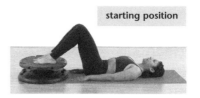
starting position

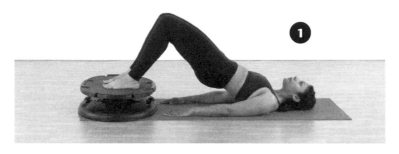
1

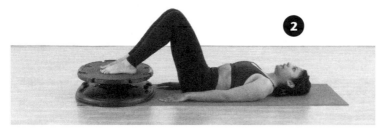
2

1 Simultaneously lift your hips and torso off the floor so that only your upper back, shoulders, and head rest on the floor. Align your shoulders and pelvis so they form one line. Plant your heels into the center of your balance board for stability and engage your buttocks to lift from your pelvis. Hold for 5 to 8 breaths.

2 Slowly lower your spine to the floor with control.

Repeat the lift 5 to 8 times.

INTERMEDIATE: Once you raise your hips, straighten your right leg, reaching from your toes. Focus on keeping your hips even and your pelvis stable as you lift your leg (the tendency is for one hip to droop). Breathe normally.

ADVANCED: Once you raise your hips, straighten your right leg. Inhale to kick the leg to the ceiling and exhale to lower it.

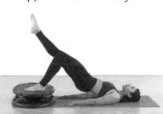

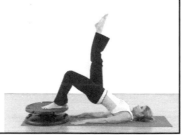

TIPS

• Engage your core muscles by exhaling deeply to create brace-like support for your torso.

plank twist on balance board

Benefits: Strengthens your core muscles, especially abdominal obliques, while challenging your total body stability

Caution: If you have a shoulder, neck, or back injury, don't do this exercise.

STARTING POSITION: Kneel in front of your balance board and place your hands on it. Walk your hips away from the board so you can get into a plank position on your knees. Lower your hips so they are in line with your torso. Inhale to find your focus.

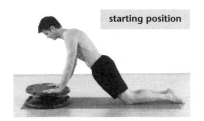

starting position

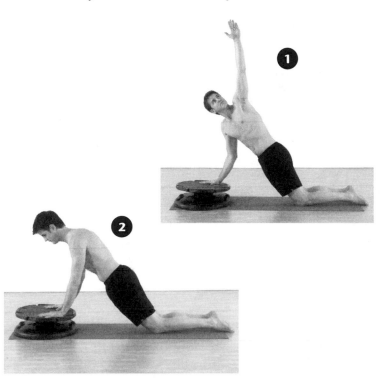

1 In one movement, exhale to lift your left arm to the ceiling and twist at the waist so your arm and fingers reach to the ceiling. Rotate from the bottom rib cage, not your lower back. Make sure your hips remain even and pointed down toward the floor.

2 Lower back to starting position.

Repeat this rotation 5 times and then switch sides.

TIPS

- Don't hike your shoulders to your ears.
- Engage your core by lifting your abs to your spine to support your lower back.
- If you experience lower back strain, first check your alignment—perhaps you're not pulling your navel to your spine. If the pain persists, then stop this exercise.
- Don't drop your head—keep it in line with your spine.

ADVANCED: To increase the challenge, do this from a plank position, keeping your legs straight.

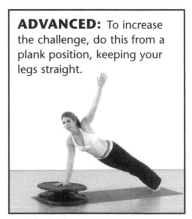

push-up on BOSU

Benefits: Strengthens your chest muscles while challenging your total body stability

This is a very advanced exercise.

STARTING POSITION: Flip the BOSU over so that the bubble end is down. Place your hands on the handles. Walk your legs out so you're in a plank position.

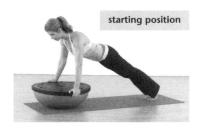

starting position

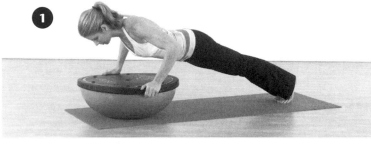

1 To a count of four, maintain your plank as you inhale to bend your elbows, lowering your nose to the BOSU.

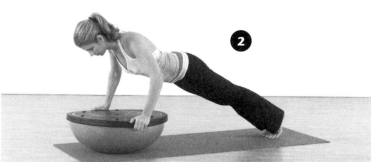

2 To a count of four, exhale to push up until your body is back in a plank position.

Repeat 5 to 8 times.

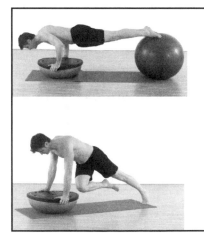

BEGINNER: If you feel very wobbly, drop to your knees.

ADVANCED: If this exercise is too easy, elevate your feet on a solid surface, such as a coffee table, or put your feet on a ball.

EXTREME: For a super-extreme challenge, in plank position, exhale to move your right knee to your left shoulder. Repeat on the other side.

Benefits: Strengthens the muscles of the leg, ankles, and feet while challenging your total body stability

This is a very advanced exercise.

STARTING POSITION: Flip the BOSU over so the bubble end is down.

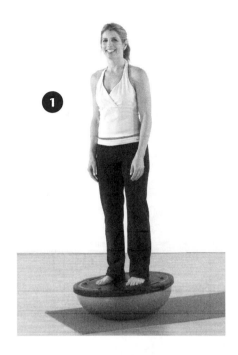

1 Stand on the BOSU with your feet a little wider than hip-width apart. You can hold your arms out to your sides for balance. Hold for 30–60 seconds.

MODIFICATION: If you feel very wobbly, use the wall for support.

BICEPS CURL VARIATION: Hold a pair of 8 or 10lb. dumbbells. When you are steady, inhale to straighten your arms by your sides and then exhale to bend your elbows to curl the dumbbells. Repeat 5 to 8 times. If this is too easy, increase the weight of the dumbbells.

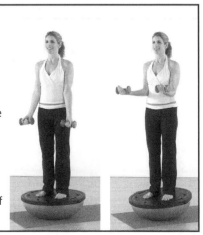

one-legged stand on BOSU

Benefits: Strengthens the muscles of the leg, ankles, and feet while challenging your total body stability

STARTING POSITION: Stand with your left foot on top of your BOSU while your right foot is placed on the floor for support.

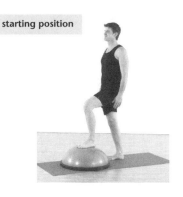

starting position

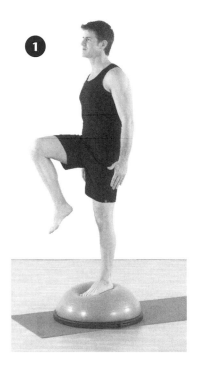

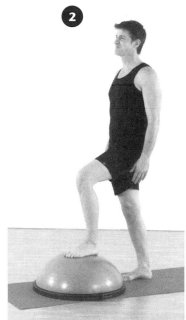

1 Shift your weight to your left leg, positioning your hip over your left foot, as you raise your right foot up and away from the floor. Engage your abdominals to maintain proper neutral spine alignment as well as keep you steady; maintain spinal stability by lifting your breastbone to help lengthen and lift your spine. Breathing normally, hold for 30 seconds.

2 Lower your right leg to the floor.

Switch legs.

MODIFICATIONS
- If you feel very wobbly, use the wall for support.
- If this exercise is too easy, close your eyes.

one-legged squat on BOSU

Benefits: Strengthens all the muscles of your legs, ankles, and feet; develops core and hip stability

STARTING POSITION: Stand with your left foot on top of your BOSU while your right foot is placed on the floor to the side in a squat position. Bend your left knee slowly to about a 90-degree angle, making sure your knee tracks over your two middle toes for proper knee alignment. Breathe normally throughout this exercise.

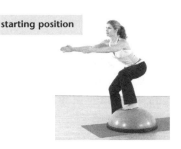

starting position

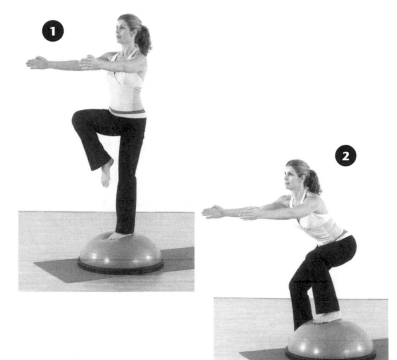

1 Shift your weight to your left leg, positioning your hip over your left foot, as you raise your right foot up and away from the floor. Maintain spinal stability by lifting your breastbone to help lengthen and lift your spine.

2 Bend your left knee slowly to about a 90-degree angle, making sure your knee tracks over your two middle toes for proper knee alignment. Sit in your heel—don't let your knee move past your toes.

3 Straighten up and balance as in step 1.

Repeat 5 to 8 times and then switch legs.

MODIFICATION
• If you feel too wobbly, use the wall for support.

one-legged lunge with leg lift on BOSU

Benefits: Strengthens all the muscles of your legs, ankles, and feet; develops core and hip stability

STARTING POSITION: Stand with your right foot on top of your BOSU while your left foot is on the floor, about two feet behind you, in a lunge position.

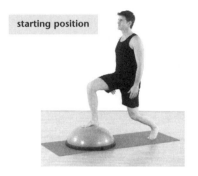

starting position

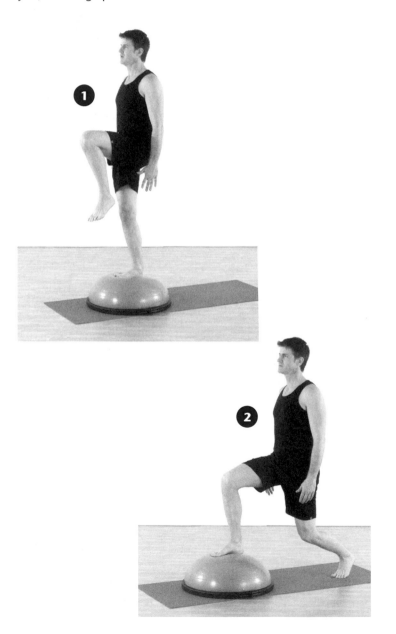

1 Simultaneously shift your weight to your right leg, positioning your hip over your right foot, as you lift your left foot off the ground, bending your knee to a 90-degree angle. Move slowly, making sure your knee is in alignment with your two middle toes. Sit into your heel—don't let your knee move past your toes. Maintain spinal stability by lifting your breastbone to help lengthen and lift your spine.

2 Return to starting position.

Repeat 5 to 8 times and then switch legs.

MODIFICATION
- If you feel too wobbly, try to lift your left knee just halfway, or use the wall for support.

one-legged deadlift on balance board

Benefits: Strengthens all the muscles of your legs, ankles, and feet; develops core and hip stability. Big bonus: Focuses on strengthening your hamstrings.

This is an extreme exercise.

STARTING POSITION: Turn the balance board lengthwise and then stand on it, placing your left foot in the middle while your right foot slightly touches the board. Maintain spinal stability by lifting your breastbone to help lengthen and lift your spine. Place your hands on your hips. Gaze at a fixed spot in front of you.

starting position

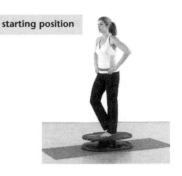

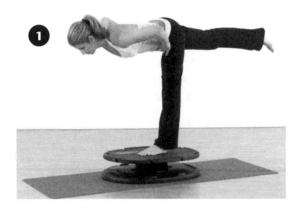

1 Slowly inhale to lift your right leg behind you, lifting from your heel to engage the buttocks and hamstrings, as you lower your torso to the ground. Your torso and leg should be in a straight line and parallel to the floor, and your hip points should be even and face down.

2 Slowly exhale to return to starting position.

Repeat 5 to 8 times and then switch legs.

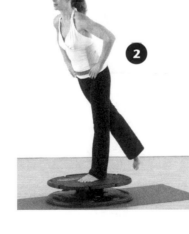

VARIATION WITH WEIGHTS: To increase the challenge, hold a pair of 8 or 10lbs dumbbell weights. Slowly lift your left leg and your right arm as your torso lowers to the ground. You can start with less weight if this is too difficult.

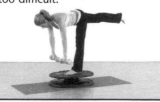

TIPS

• Engage your core muscles to help you stabilize and keep your hips even.

half moon

Benefits: Strengthens all the muscles of your legs, ankles, and feet; develops core and hip stability. Big bonus: Focuses on strengthening your hamstrings.

STARTING POSITION: Turn the balance board lengthwise and then stand on it, placing your left foot in the middle while your right foot slightly touches the board. Maintain spinal stability by lifting your breastbone to help lengthen and lift your spine. Gaze at a fixed spot in front of you.

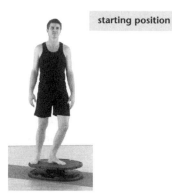
starting position

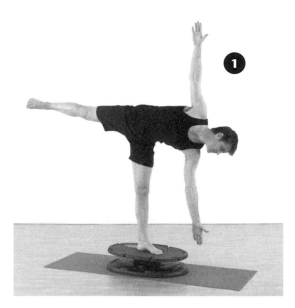

1 Slowly inhale to lift your leg to the side, lifting from your heel to engage the buttocks and hamstrings as you lower your torso to the ground. Your torso and leg should be in a straight line out to the side. Your hips points should be stacked on top of one another. Open your chest to the side and lift one arm to the ceiling and the other to the floor; your arms should create a straight line. Look down.

ADVANCED: To increase the challenge, you can also look up to the ceiling.

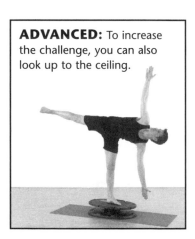

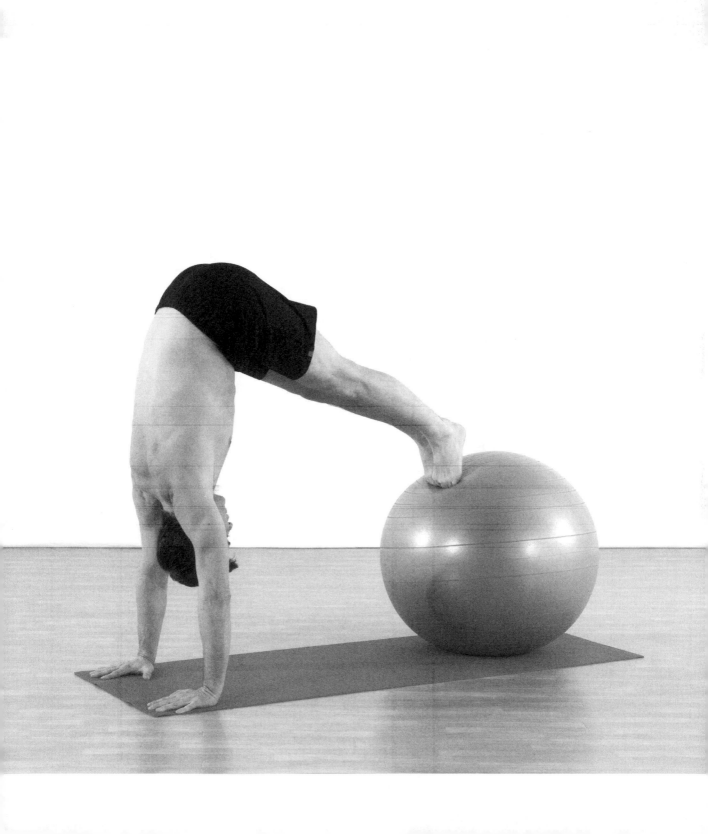

index

other ulysses press books

BELLY DANCING FOR FITNESS: THE ULTIMATE DANCE WORKOUT THAT UNLEASHES YOUR CREATIVE SPIRIT
Tamalyn Dallal with Richard Harris, $14.95

A healthy aerobic workout that adds dancing, exotic music, the twirl of silk and the rhythmic clanging of finger cymbals.

ELLIE HERMAN'S PILATES MATWORK PROPS WORKBOOK:STEP-BY-STEP GUIDE WITH OVER 200 PHOTOS
Ellie Herman, $15.95

Explains how props such as the magic circle, small ball, foam roller and balance ball can enhance Pilates.

ELLIE HERMAN'S PILATES WORKBOOK ON THE BALL: ILLUSTRATED STEP-BY-STEP GUIDE
Ellie Herman, $14.95

Combines the powerful slimming and shaping effects of Pilates with the low-impact, high-intensity workout of the ball.

FIT IN 15: 15-MINUTE MORNING WORKOUTS THAT BALANCE CARDIO, STRENGTH AND FLEXIBILITY
Steven Stiefel, $12.95

Fit in 15 details a unique, full-body fitness program that even the busiest person can work into a morning schedule.

FORZA: THE SAMURAI SWORD WORKOUT
Ilaria Montagnani, $14.95

Transforms sword-fighting techniques into a program that combines the excitement of sword play with a heart-pumping, full-body workout.

FUNCTIONAL TRAINING FOR ATHLETES AT ALL LEVELS: WORKOUTS FOR AGILITY, SPEED AND POWER
James C. Radcliffe, $15.95

Teaches athletes the exercises that will produce the best results in their sport by mimicking the actual movements they utilized in that sport.

THE MARTIAL ARTIST'S BOOK OF YOGA
Lily Chou with Kathe Rothacher, $14.95

A great training supplement for martial artists, this book illustrates how specific yoga poses can directly improve one's martial arts abilities.

PILATES WORKBOOK: ILLUSTRATED STEP-BY-STEP GUIDE TO MATWORK TECHNIQUES
Michael King, $12.95

Illustrates the core matwork movements exactly as Joseph Pilates intended them to be performed.

PLYOMETRICS FOR ATHLETES AT ALL LEVELS: A TRAINING GUIDE FOR EXPLOSIVE SPEED AND POWER
Neal Pire, $15.95

Provides an easy-to-understand explanation of why plyometrics works, the research behind it, and how to integrate it into a fitness program.

TOTAL HEART RATE TRAINING: CUSTOMIZE AND MAXIMIZE YOUR WORKOUT USING A HEART RATE MONITOR
Joe Friel, $14.95

Shows anyone participating in aerobic sports how to increase the effectiveness of his or her workout by utilizing a heart rate monitor.

WEIGHT-BEARING WORKOUTS FOR WOMEN: EXERCISES FOR SCULPTING, STRENGTHENING & TONING
Yolande Green, $12.95

Weight training is the most effective way to lose fat, improve muscle tone and strengthen bones. This workbook shows just how easy it is for women at any age to get started with weights.

WEIGHTS FOR 50+: BUILDING STRENGTH, STAYING HEALTHY AND ENJOYING AN ACTIVE LIFESTYLE
Dr. Karl Knopf, $14.95

Shows how easy it is for a 50+ person to lift weights, stay fit and active, and guard against osteoporosis, diabetes and heart disease.

WEIGHTS ON THE BALL WORKBOOK: STEP-BY-STEP GUIDE WITH OVER 350 PHOTOS
Steven Stiefel, $14.95

With exercises suited for all skill levels, *Weights on the Ball Workbook* shows how to simultaneously use weights and the exercise ball for the ultimate total-body workout.

WORKOUTS FROM BOXING'S GREATEST CHAMPS
Gary Todd, $14.95

Features dramatic photos, workout secrets and behind-the-scenes details of Muhammad Ali, Roy Jones, Jr., Fernando Vargas and other legends.

To order these books call 800-377-2542 or 510-601-8301, fax 510-601-8307, e-mail ulysses@ ulyssespress.com, or write to Ulysses Press, P.O. Box 3440, Berkeley, CA 94703. All retail orders are shipped free of charge. California residents must include sales tax. Allow two to three weeks for delivery.

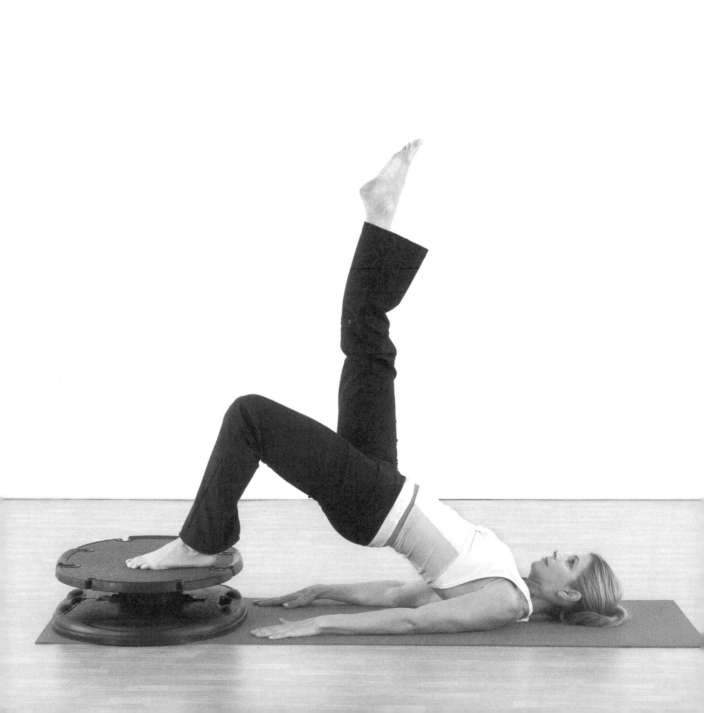

about the author

KARON KARTER has 15 years' experience in the fitness and health industry, and is trained in Pilates, Resist-a-Ball and Ashtanga yoga. Her health and fitness books (*The Complete Idiot's Guide to Body Ball Illustrated, The Core Strength Workout, The Complete Idiot's Guide to Pilates, The Complete Idiot's Guide to Kickboxing, The Healthy Flier*) have sold over 150,000 copies; her most recent publication, *Pilates Lite,* appears in five languages. Karon has been featured in the *New York Times,* the *Miami Herald,* the *Dallas Morning News* and other major newspapers, and writes health and fitness articles for *D-Magazine,* the *Dallas Morning News* and *PilatesStyle* magazine. She can also be seen on television as the host of *Pilates From the Inside Out!* Karon teaches classes at her Pilates studio in Dallas, Texas.

about the photographer

ANDY MOGG is a well-known and much-published photographer. Born in England in 1954, he worked as a consultant, then writer and photographer. At 17, he moved from London to Belgium, traveling and working his way through Europe; he settled in the United States 20 years ago. He now runs a thriving photography studio in Oakland, California. For more information, visit his website at www.dancingimages.com.